Living with Max

To Wiesia

Happy Birthday!

Living with Max

Hope you enjoy!

[signature]

xoxo

CHLOE MAXWELL

For every copy of this book sold in Australia and
New Zealand, the author and publisher are making a
donation to 4ASD Kids, a charity which helps children who
have Autism Spectrum Disorder and their families.

HarperCollins*Publishers*

HarperCollins*Publishers*

First published in Australia in 2012
by HarperCollins*Publishers* Australia Pty Limited
ABN 36 009 913 517
harpercollins.com.au

Text copyright © Chloe Maxwell 2012

HarperCollins*Publishers*
Level 13, 201 Elizabeth Street, Sydney NSW 2000, Australia
31 View Road, Glenfield, Auckland 0627, New Zealand
A 53, Sector 57, Noida, UP, India
77–85 Fulham Palace Road, London, W6 8JB, United Kingdom
2 Bloor Street East, 20th floor, Toronto, Ontario M4W 1A8, Canada
10 East 53rd Street, New York NY 10022, USA
National Library of Australia Cataloguing-in-Publication entry

Maxwell, Chloe.
  Living with Max : our family story / Chloe Maxwell.
  978 0 7322 9228 7 (pbk.)
  Maxwell, Chloe.
  Rogers, Max.
  Rogers family.
  Autistic children – Australia – Biography.
  Children with autism spectrum disorders – Australia.
  Parents of autistic children – Australia – Biography.
616.858820092

Cover design by Jane Waterhouse, HarperCollins Design Studio
Cover photography by Stuart Scott
Typeset in 11.5/18pt Adobe Caslon by Kirby Jones
Printed and bound in Australia by Griffin Press
The papers used by HarperCollins in the manufacture of this book are a natural,
recyclable product made from wood grown in sustainable plantation forests. The fibre
source and manufacturing processes meet recognised international environmental
standards, and carry certification.

5 4 3 2 1   12 13 14 15

I would like to dedicate this book to my amazing husband, who is my safe haven when it storms; my parents Michael and Di and my stepparents Ross and Jo, whom I grow to love and understand more and more each day; my incredibly talented brother and sister, Brodie and Camilla; my friends who were there to dry my tears — you know who you are; my stepkids Jack and Skyla; my daughter Phoenix, and of course my brave little soldier Max.

I hope I make you proud.

Preface

I have been blessed with an amazing life. If I have discovered only one thing through it all so far, it is that there will always be obstacles on your journey to self-discovery that will test you — and teach you, if you let them. There is always a price to pay for blessings, though.

My son has been the trigger for so much learning and healing. He may be autistic to others but to me he is a gift from God, sent to teach me to become a better parent and a better person. Nobody is perfect and I am far from it, but I do strive to be better every day. And in the midst of it all, Max reminds me that you don't have to be perfect to be a precious part of this world.

I know that in reading this book, many who are close to me will feel old wounds begin to open again. I can only hope that their understanding stretches beyond these words to see the benefit this story may have to others who suffer in the same circumstances.

As a teenager I loved poetry; W.B. Yeats was one of my favourite poets. He was never afraid to show the sordid side, the real side of life. So many other poets of his era wrote of beauty and perfection that is apparent to the eye, whereas Yeats showed what lay beyond physical beauty and external perfection, the deeper reality that exists beneath. I've chosen some fragments of his work to illuminate my story in a way that my own words could not.

1

Turning and turning in the widening gyre
The falcon cannot hear the falconer;
Things fall apart; the centre cannot hold …

— W.B. Yeats, 'The Second Coming'

Beads of sweat moistened my palms as my heartbeat pounded out the seconds. Everything else in the world was still. I waited for the man across the desk to speak.

I looked at he who would change my life forever, and wondered how many other people he had given this news to in his working life. This week. Today.

Slowly, a little casually, the doctor handed me a piece of paper. Just a single sheet: it seemed strange that something so light and innocent could cause so much turmoil. The words on that sheet were heavy, though, so heavy they made my fingers numb. Suddenly clumsy, I fumbled with it. My eyes scanned the lines of text until they found the letters I was so much hoping would not be there.

A. S. D.

My voice disappeared for a moment, swallowed down to somewhere in the region of my stomach. Then it returned, shaky and uncertain.

'S-so my son has an — an ASD. What — what does that mean, exactly?' I asked.

I knew what it meant. For the past month I had read case study after case study on the internet, devouring facts, theories and stories on the subject.

'Autism spectrum disorder,' the doctor said. His voice was metallic, robotic, as if he had been programmed to give me this diagnosis. He was our family paediatrician, but I had only visited him twice before, so he was a stranger to me.

I sat silently, imploring him with my eyes for something else. I wanted a 'but': 'But your son's case is different.'

No buts were forthcoming. 'It can mean anything from being a brain dead mute to an absolute genius.' Did he really just say that?

'Einstein had Asperger's, which is part of the spectrum. So did Mozart, they believe,' he went on.

'That's great, Doctor. But will my son play sport? Will he get married? Will he look me in the eye? Will he ever be able to say, "Where's Daddy?" or "I love you, Mummy"? Will he? WILL HE?' I saw myself leap across the desk, wrapping my hands around the doctor's robot throat and squeezing until his tongue hung limp from his mouth.

4

Still seated but raging inside, I forced myself to look away, to the ranks of toy dinosaurs lining the window ledge and the desk. I felt like ripping the office apart, a velociraptor on the rampage.

Max's scream broke me out of my murderous fantasies. Sensing my withdrawal, the doctor had taken Max to stand on the scales in the next room. Max was not happy about this. It was always this way: he simply could not understand the most trivial task or request, and he would respond by freaking out to the point of violence. Towards others, and sometimes to himself.

I dashed over to help. Max was writhing like a mad child; when I wrapped my arms around him, he managed to drive a fingernail deep into my arm, drawing blood. The doctor struggled through the process of taking his measurements, with Max spitting violently on the floor between his screams. Then it was all over. Pat-on-the-back-and-pay-the-bill time.

It's just his job, it's not his fault, I told myself as we walked out to the car. But I was still reeling from the impact of those three letters. ASD.

The thing was, I had already told my family weeks earlier that Max was autistic.

2

A mouth that has no moisture and no breath
Breathless mouths may summon …

— W.B. Yeats, 'Byzantium'

When I was sixteen years old, I became a model. Even my 'discovery' was a public event: Ursula Hufnagl, the head of Chic Management, was doing a story with *A Current Affair* on how she could pick girls off the street and make them into models, and as part of the story they found me.

It was the September school holidays. I was walking through Pitt Street Mall in Sydney, heading back to my dad's office after running an errand for him. I spotted the camera crew before they spotted me, so I made an extra effort to do my best 'model walk', strutting along to get their attention. Ursula turned and saw me then gestured to the crew to follow as she rushed towards me with a microphone in her hand. After they interviewed me in the middle of the busy mall, Ursula gave me her card and asked me to get my parents to ring her. The following week I went along to a studio in Surry Hills for a fashion shoot — and just like that, my new career was up and running.

The day Ursula discovered me, I had no real aspirations to be a model. Years earlier my mother had sent my pictures to an agency; they said I was not model material. So when Ursula asked me on national TV if I would like to be one, I had no expectations and nothing to lose. 'Sure, if you want to pay me I'll do it,' I said.

Thanks to the publicity on *A Current Affair*, my first few modelling jobs were *Vogue Australia* fashion spreads and an Esprit campaign shot in Fiji. My world would never be the same again.

While I was taking my first steps in the modelling world, the future love of my life and father of my children was playing rugby union at The Southport School in Queensland. Mat Rogers' father Steve had been captain of Australia's rugby league team and a star player for the Cronulla Sharks. With those genes and his own natural talent, Mat's destiny was assured. Back then though, both of us were just starting out, our trajectories quite unconnected.

Although I was working as a model with all of the top photographers in Australia, I was still a schoolgirl. Mum or Dad would drop me off for shoots after school. I would get out of my shabby school uniform, put on a two thousand dollar dress and glam it up. When the shoot was finished I would hang up the designer dress and put my uniform back on, still with full hair and makeup.

By nights and on the weekends I was forging an exciting career for myself. By day, however, I was living a nightmare. I was in Year 9 at Roseville Ladies College on Sydney's North Shore. It was a private school for 'ladies', apparently; however, I struggled to see anyone who could be called a lady there. Particularly among one group of girls, who had decided that I was the person to pick on.

'Heidi doesn't like you and she wants to bash you, she told me to tell you,' an unknown Year 10 girl with a lopsided grin spat at me as I was walking to maths one morning.

'What? Who's Heidi? I don't even know her,' I squeaked as she turned on her heel and stalked off down the hallway.

'Scrag!' A nasal yell rang out across the playground as I stood in line at the tuckshop. I pretended I didn't realise it was directed at me, but from the corner of my eye I saw a group of older girls snickering at me. These were not your average girls, I must say. Had I not been at an all-girls school I would have questioned the gender of at least one of them. After they threatened to fight anyone who hung out with me, my group of friends began to diminish.

When another student asked them why they had decided to pick on me, they answered, 'Because she always wears her hair on the side and she never smiles.' After I heard that I became a smiling idiot who never wore her hair on the side. Didn't stop the taunting though.

Often I would come home from school crying. I would have

nightmares of being beaten to death in a park by these girls, left naked and flecked with their spit.

Things got worse when my modelling career took off at the end of Year 9. I counted down the days until the bullies would finish school and be out of my life for good. Eventually they completed Year 12, and I was able to start enjoying school once more.

Years later when I was a VJ (video jockey) on Channel V, I came face to face with those girls again. One came up to me when I was shooting a dance music show in Wollongong, and I had to interview another who was part of a manufactured reality TV pop group. They apologised to me for what they had put me through in high school.

For me, the bully girls always gave me just one more reason to succeed.

During my school years we lived in a cul-de-sac in Wahroonga, a beautiful outer suburb of Sydney. Our home was a big old two-storey house surrounded by bushland. My brother, sister and I moved there with Mum and her boyfriend Ross (whom she later married) after my mum and dad separated. I was fourteen, and all of a sudden my father was just not there. After seventeen years of marriage, my parents had both found new life partners. They were moving on, but kids take a little longer to come to terms with these things.

My mother is a beautiful woman with strawberry blonde hair like my sister Camilla, but her features are more like mine. At that time in our lives, she had suffered a lot: in quick succession, finding out her husband was perhaps being unfaithful and then losing her father to lung cancer. She had a grey hair for every one of those life lessons, she would tell me, but nothing that a regular visit to the hairdresser wouldn't fix. In those early days she always managed to have a positive and almost light-hearted attitude toward adversity.

I remember driving her home from Christmas drinks one year — this was a few years after Mum and Dad separated, when I was in my twenties. We were turning right at a set of lights in Manly when a P-plater came flying straight through the intersection against a red light. The air bags in my brand-new Honda Prelude exploded out of the dashboard and part of the panel lacerated her eye. It was a horrific injury: her eye looked as though it was hanging out of her head. But after the ambulance came she was laughing with the paramedics and cracking jokes. I admired her so much for being able to do that. The few champagnes she'd had might have gone a long way to help, but even the next day at the hospital she was joking around with the doctors. She would say to one, 'My husband told me he shouldn't have to ask me twice.' And to another, 'You should see the other guy!' and she would throw back her head and let out her deep guttural laugh, despite the obvious seriousness of the situation.

I suspect I was a horrible big sister. When we were growing up I was an absolute bitch to my brother and sister, and I used to play tricks on them all the time. I was always showing off, wanting to be the centre of attention and bossing people around. I'd make my brother and sister act in my plays: they had to dress up, and I'd direct the play — so they had to do what I said. My brother was inevitably dressed up as a girl, and if he tried to get out of his costume, I'd yell at him: 'Put that back on and get out and do your lines.'

In our teenage years, we became closer. After our parents divorced, we banded together more: endlessly moving between two houses, we were the only constant in each others' lives, in a way.

My sister Camilla is five years younger than me. We don't look very much alike: she has fine features, beautiful porcelain skin and that strawberry blonde hair. When I was in my last year of high school, I came home from school one day to find Camilla on the phone, shivering as she spoke softly into the receiver.

'What are you doing?' I asked. She ignored me and kept whispering into the phone. I dropped my schoolbag on the floor and poked my tongue out at the back of her head. She really got on my nerves sometimes, as little sisters can.

I walked into the kitchen and opened the fridge, looking for something to snack on before Mum came home from work and cooked dinner. Us kids would often be home before her, since she worked long hours as a legal secretary in the city. Mum's boyfriend Ross was a barrister and also her boss. Neither of them would be home for another couple of hours, and my brother Brodie was at basketball, so it was just Camilla and me in the house.

As I shut the fridge door my sister appeared. She looked quite green and pretty shaken up.

'Dad's on the phone, he wants to speak to you,' she croaked, sounding hung-over or ill. I was used to Camilla over-dramatising when she was sick. Often she would wrap bandages around her wrists or legs, feigning injury. Looking back I think she was deeply affected by our parents' separation and desperate for some attention.

I went into the other room and picked up the receiver.

'Hi, Dad,' I said cheerfully.

'Chloe, something very serious is happening,' he said in a tone of voice I had never heard him use before.

'What's wrong?' I asked, puzzled but with an edge of sarcasm in my voice too, thinking that my sister had dreamt up yet another way of getting attention.

'Now don't panic, but Camilla has just swallowed a whole box of Panadol to try to kill herself. I need you to take her to Emergency right away.'

My heart skipped a beat. I stretched the phone cord so I could lean back to look at Camilla. She had collapsed on the couch and was breathing very irregularly.

'What?' I asked, thinking this was some sort of joke. 'Why did she call you then?'

'She decided she didn't want to die and called me for help, Chloe. Now get her in the car and drive!' He sounded close to tears.

'OK!' I hung up the receiver, grabbed my keys and tried to help Camilla to her feet. She was not in a good way.

'What were you thinking, Camilla?' I suddenly felt anger burning in my throat. She didn't reply. Dragging her outside, I managed to prop her up in the passenger seat of my little Mazda 323. I had only recently got my licence and I was still not one hundred per cent confident with passengers. No time to think about that now. I pushed her head back onto the headrest and slipped the seat belt around her.

I sped all the way to the hospital in a state of panic. Camilla looked so calm in the passenger seat, but she was drifting in and out of consciousness. We made it to Emergency, where Camilla had to have her stomach pumped.

'She had definitely swallowed those pills,' the nurse assured me as I watched her lie sleeping on a hospital bed. A white curtain separated us from the rest of the casualties that surrounded us. I wondered how many other suicide attempts were being rectified out there right now.

Mum finally arrived and launched herself at the bed. 'Oh my God, Camilla,' she whimpered. I imagined several more grey hairs appearing on her head.

We discovered later that Camilla had been suffering at the hands of bullies at school. She was getting a dose of the same hostility I had faced, but in her case the other girls were taunting her with my success, saying things like, 'Your sister is a model, so how come you are so ugly?' My beautiful little sister had begun to believe all of the horrible things they were saying about her. Put that together with the fact that she blamed herself for our parents' marriage collapsing, and her emotions had simply reached breaking point.

After changing schools, Camilla found a new confidence — both in her later school years and beyond. Ironically perhaps, she has now forged a successful path in the acting world. Most importantly, she has never tried to take her own life again.

I see success as the sweetest revenge for bullying. I certainly gained mental toughness through my teen years — from my torment at school, the fragmentation of my family and my work as a model, too. Working with some of the biggest names in fashion, I experienced both the high life of the fashion industry and the dirty underbelly. Being a model, you can't help but grow up pretty quickly.

While I was travelling the world, appearing on the pages of international fashion magazines, my husband-to-be was steadily gaining a name for himself as an incredibly gifted football player, representing Australia in rugby union and rugby league — a 'dual code international' they call it. Even so, when we first met I didn't know who he was, and he didn't know who I was either. I think that was what we liked so much about each other.

3

O body swayed to music, O brightening glance,
How can we know the dancer from the dance?

— W.B. Yeats, 'Among School Children'

Modelling morphed into television presenting and then in
November 2004, the dream job came my way. A new talent show,
The X Factor, needed a host, and after four years as a VJ on Channel
V I couldn't wait to get into free to air. This was where it was at,
career-wise and money-wise. *The X Factor* was huge in the UK, and
Channel Ten were hoping to replicate that success here in Australia.
Daniel MacPherson, well known from his roles in *Neighbours* and
the legendary UK series *The Bill*, was the host and I would be his
co-host, presenting the behind-the-scenes show *The Xtra Factor*.

It was exactly what I had been working towards, but there
was just one glitch that could spoil this rosy picture. Filming was
due to start on the Monday. On the Saturday night, my then-
boyfriend and (I thought) the love of my life decided it would be
a great idea to hit on my sister.

We had gone out for dinner and dancing to celebrate my brother's birthday. My dad had come too and it was quite a novelty to have him dancing and drinking with us in the hot spots of Sydney's Oxford Street. I spent most of the night dancing with Dad. I had a fantastic night and had no idea about anything untoward until the following morning.

I had just jumped in the shower to rinse away my hangover when I heard soft murmurings coming from the garden. It was my boyfriend, talking to someone on the phone.

I thought nothing of it and went on getting ready for the day. Then my phone rang. It was Camilla and I could tell from her voice that she was very upset.

'Chloe, I wanted to let you know about someone's behaviour that I just don't agree with.' She was trembling so much I could hear the phone shaking. Camilla went on to tell me that my boyfriend had been trying to convince her to have a relationship with him behind my back. While I was in the shower, she had called to give him a piece of her mind, and apparently he was trying to convince her not to say anything to me so that they could see each other without me knowing. He was delusional.

I got off the phone and flew into a rage. I kicked his backside out of my house then drove to my mum's place, where I drowned my sorrows in several bottles of wine.

Next morning I arrived at Homebush for the first day of filming. Smelling of alcohol from the night before and with red swollen eyes from the many tears I had shed — and was still shedding, even though there couldn't possibly be any moisture left in my tear ducts — I sheepishly sidled past the crew unloading equipment from vans. I bumped into one of the runners near the stadium entrance and she showed me through to a storage room in the depths of the stadium, where I was to wait for Daniel and the producer. I collapsed on a chair and fell asleep, emotionally exhausted.

'Maxwell? C-Max?'

I awoke to Daniel's voice. My swollen lids slowly forced themselves open.

'Oh my God! What the hell happened to you?' He lifted my dark glasses off my face, genuine concern in his green eyes.

I dumped all the gory details on him as we shared a cigarette. He was very understanding and quite charming, brushing the hair from my cheek and nodding all the while. I wondered if we would ever be more than friends. He was a lot shorter than me.

Australia Day 2005: After shooting *The X Factor* auditions for a couple of months, we were due to move to Melbourne that day to finish off the auditions and remain there for the live shows. Before we flew out in the afternoon, the network had invited Daniel and me to be their guests in the Channel Ten VIP marquee for an Australia Day party at Randwick Racecourse.

Daniel had brought his dad 'Macca' along. The two of them had both recently become bachelors and were regularly going out together, which I thought was very cute. Daniel's dad seemed to be great value, just as cheeky as his son, so I knew I was in for a fun day.

The Channel Ten marquee was right by the finish line; it also happened to be next door to the marquee for the New South Wales Waratahs — the state's rugby union team. This tent was distinguished by the stocky men in suits with thick necks and cauliflower ears milling around in front of it.

Daniel was originally from Cronulla and loved his footy, so he was familiar with all the guys in this tent. I was completely clueless. My weekends had been spent in nightclubs and at raves and outdoor dance parties; I had never been interested in footy and today was no different. I was, however, interested in drinking free champagne. It was what I was using to fill the void where my ex-boyfriend had been.

That morning I had decided to wear one of the biggest hats I could find to hide under, as I knew the champagne would be on tap all day. I had also chosen a bright red figure-hugging dress — being newly single, it had to be tight. I sauntered to the bar to get us drinks, revelling in any male attention I could get along the way. When I returned a burly-looking guy was sitting with Daniel, laughing and chatting. He was obviously from the tent next door, and although he didn't fit the criteria of what I usually looked for in a guy, there was something about him.

'Maxwell?' Daniel called me by my last name all the time; I think it's a private school thing.

'Chloe Maxwell, this is Mat Rogers. Mat, Chloe.' Daniel gestured between us with a cold beer in his hand.

'How ya going?' I asked rather yobbishly and slid between them at the table, clutching my ridiculously huge hat while simultaneously lighting a cigarette.

'Oh, I'm hanging out for one of those,' Mat said, looking at me hungrily.

'Really?' I replied in a cat-like purr.

'Yeah, I can't smoke while the coach is here though.'

My face flooded with crimson as I took an extra-long drag on my ciggie and gulped down some more French champagne.

'So do you play football or something?' I asked, trying to keep the conversation rolling.

Daniel and his dad broke out into fits of laughter.

'Um, only for Australia, Maxwell!' Daniel might have been good-looking but he was fast getting on my nerves.

'Oh,' I said. 'Sorry, I don't watch football.' I shifted uncomfortably in my seat. It was really hot and the combination of embarrassment and too much champagne was beginning to make me perspire. The last thing I wanted was a sweat mark on the back of my dress.

'How can you smoke and play footy?' I asked, finding my spunk again.

'I guess I was just blessed with some talent,' he said.

Now that made me want to gag. Has this bloke got tickets on himself or what? I thought. Oh well, I'm here to have fun, I reminded myself, so I may as well flirt with him. The urge to gag subsided — for now.

'Daniel says you're working with him on a TV show — what doing?' Mat asked, maybe sensing how badly received his last comment was.

'She's my co-host with the mo-ost!' Daniel sang. This boy was born to be on TV. He had a knack for sounding as though he was presenting, even in normal conversation.

Mat looked confused.

'Chloe Maxwell — you know, she was on Channel V,' Daniel explained.

'Sorry … were you on Channel V?' Mat asked.

I nodded, taking a big drag on my cigarette and blowing smoke in his face.

The rest of the day was spent talking about our exes and making fun of all the punters milling around us and basking in their own importance. These tents were pretty exclusive and most of the people in them knew that — and it showed. It was fantastic people-watching fodder.

Mat told me he had broken up with his wife and was living in a serviced apartment in a hotel in Darling Harbour. His two kids, Jack and Skyla, stayed with him there on the weekends.

I relived with him my still-fresh injury at the hands of my ex and we proceeded to drown our sorrows together. I fast discovered that I had met my match when it came to drinking alcohol and holding it together. I was impressed. Some might say too easily.

Midway through our mutual commiseration session, a lady dressed in a bright green frock tapped me on the shoulder.

'Excuse me, Chloe, you have made it into the final of Fashions on the Field.' By this stage I had probably drunk my own body weight in champagne, so I began to giggle uncontrollably at the amazing resemblance her fascinator bore to Gordon, my old pet budgie.

'If you wouldn't mind making your way to the stage in the Channel Ten marquee at 2 p.m. on the dot. The winner will be decided by cheers from the audience.' Clearly agitated by my lack of enthusiasm, she spun on her heel and little Gordon flew away. I followed him with my eyes for a short time and then I turned back to the boys.

'Right, if I'm going to do this I need your support.' I gestured at them with my half-empty glass of champagne.

All three of the boys nodded. 'We'll come cheer you on, Maxwell,' Daniel exclaimed as he and Mat began studying the racing guide intently.

Two o'clock rolled around and I had pretty much forgotten that I was supposed to be up at the stage. We had shared so many funny stories, my sides were sore from laughing — or maybe my liver was kicking out in protest.

Gordon and his green perch appeared again. 'Chloe, if you wouldn't mind coming with me now. We're waiting for you,' the perch said.

'Don't forget, you guys, you have to come and cheer me on,' I slurred. The boys were still studying the form guide but they all nodded absently as Gordon and his perch led me through the crowd into the depths of the marquee.

Finally we arrived at the side of the stage. Two other girls waited anxiously there; they both looked gorgeous.

'And our finalists for Fashions on the Field are …' the MC's voice came amplified from the stage as the crowd's attention shifted to the three girls waiting in the wings. He called us up one by one. I was a little shaky getting up the steps and secretly cursed Gordon and his perch for getting me into this predicament.

The three of us stood there in our best fashion poses while the MC ran through the prizes available to the winner. I scanned the crowd, hoping this wasn't going to be as humiliating as it was starting to seem. No Daniel. No Mat.

'If he was trying to impress me, this is not working in his favour,' I thought.

It was time for the crowd to choose. The MC turned to the girl on my left. 'Who thinks contestant number one should win today?' he said as the crowd erupted into cheers and applause. The girl did a little turn then curtsied.

'Great,' I muttered under my breath. With the amount of champagne I had drunk, there was no way I would be attempting anything like that. Mind you, I had always fared pretty well at Fashion Week after a few drinks. I only fell off the end of the runway once.

'What about contestant two, who thinks she should win?' he said, gesturing at me. I put my hand on my hip and smiled and waved as best I could without swaying too much.

A single 'Yay!' was heard from the back of the room. I think it was Daniel's dad Macca, but I couldn't be sure. Daniel and Mat were nowhere to be seen.

'Hmmm — and who here thinks contestant three should win today?' The crowd erupted again.

My forced smile was beginning to waver as I pictured myself stubbing out the cigarette I was desperate to have on Daniel's and Mat's limbs. When I found them.

'OK, it appears to be a tie between contestant one and contestant three, so one more time. Contestant one' — his hand flew past my head — 'or contestant three?'

'Is this guy serious?' I thought to myself. He had left me standing up there while they did a cheer-off for the other two contestants. I felt like the biggest tool!

Finally a decision was made; the winner was given all of her wonderful prizes as we, two losers, stood and looked on.

Later I found out that in fact Daniel and Mat had been cheering very loudly. Just not for me, but for the horse they had a hundred bucks on.

4

By the dark webs, her nape caught in his bill,
He holds her helpless breast upon his breast.

— W.B. Yeats, 'Leda and the Swan'

I left the races and flew straight down to Melbourne that afternoon. This is where all of the live performances for *The X Factor* would be filmed, and it would be my home for the next three months. I came back to Sydney often, though had to be back in Melbourne for rehearsals and coaching to improve my breathing techniques for speaking and working with the autocue. Like anything, it takes a bit of work to make these things seem effortless.

The network had put me up in a cute little apartment in St Kilda. Someone who lived nearby told me it was owned by Claudia Karvan's mum, and even if it wasn't true I was stoked with that idea — maybe some of Claudia's talent would rub off on me, I thought. This show was a really big deal for me: I so much wanted to make a success of it.

The demons that attacked me daily seemed set on making me fail, though. For a while there it seemed to be a showdown between good Chloe and evil Chloe, and most days the evil one seemed to have the upper hand. Funny how the dark side prevails when you're at your most vulnerable.

I loved living in St Kilda; it was such a funky place to be. In retrospect, though, it probably wasn't the best place in the world to put someone suffering from a broken heart. I was surrounded by all of my favourite distractions — clubs, alcohol and rock 'n' roll — while working on a massive reality television production as the on-air talent. There was a lot riding on this — for me and for the producers — so I made sure I found ways to let off steam.

I enjoyed plenty of big nights out and quickly made friends with the crew members who were up for partying too. One friend from my Channel V days was singer and makeup artist Suzani Rain. She has the most gorgeous face and is covered in piercings and tattoos. At the time she was working at The Vineyard, a buzzy bar and restaurant just opposite Luna Park. Suzani is a remarkable performer. We clicked and became drinking buddies pretty quickly.

I would walk down to meet her at The Vineyard when she finished work and we would generally start drinking there. Then we would do a pub crawl and check out some bands. There's always great live music going on in Melbourne, any hour of the night or day. Most nights I would end up stumbling home in the early hours, which made getting up for work in the morning very difficult.

Not too far from where I was living was the heart of St Kilda's notorious sex trade district. I delighted in people-watching around there; in the early hours of the morning there was always something interesting going on with the prostitutes and their clients. I remember heading off for work early one morning, feeling pretty sorry for myself after a big night out. At a standstill in traffic, I looked out the window of my cab and saw a working girl looking extremely dishevelled. Her very short dress was creased and covered in stains, and her fishnet tights were ripped and laddered. She had taken one stiletto off and was holding it while balancing a cigarette on her bottom lip. She appeared to be dancing.

I wound down my window to listen for the music. Nothing. The girl was now buckled over, folded in half, her head hovering just above the ground. She seemed to be asleep standing up, but in fact she was in a state heroin addicts call 'on the nod'. It used to amaze me that junkies could stand like this with their heads inches from the ground, semiconscious.

Outlandish though she looked, I didn't find her funny. I felt sorry for her, but at the same time watching her made me somehow feel better about myself. As terrible as that sounds, it's the same impulse that makes people read trashy gossip magazines and watch bad television shows: in some weird way, seeing or reading about other people's misfortunes makes them feel better about their own lives.

As I kept watching, I was amused by the reactions of other

people passing by, ordinary men and women on their way to ordinary jobs. Most pretended the girl wasn't there; others made disapproving noises. One old lady stopped walking and bent down to say something to her; I couldn't hear the words, but the woman's face had disgust written all over it. All of a sudden, the working girl sprang to life and chased her up the street. Moving surprisingly fast on one shoe, she sped after the woman, hurling abuse and her other stiletto.

Why that woman felt the need to say something I don't know, but I'm sure she'll think twice about it next time. Who knew what had led this working girl to sell sex for drugs? More often than not there's a tale of woe behind these things. The dark side prevails when you're at your most vulnerable, after all.

It's so easy to judge people when you don't know them or their story. In Stephen Covey's book *The Seven Habits of Highly Effective People*, he recalls seeing a man on the train with his two sons. The kids are going wild, wrestling each other and bouncing off the walls as young children can do. The other passengers are clearly agitated with the kids and finally Stephen decides to say something to the father, along the lines of, 'Can't you control your children?' To which the man replies, 'We just got back from the hospital where their mother died. I don't know how to handle it, I guess.'

Once you know a little about someone's situation, it makes all the difference. Later in my life I, too, would often be approached by strangers who spoke out without having all the facts.

Mat and I spoke often on the phone after we met that day at the races. Before Daniel and I were whisked off in a limousine to the airport, Mat asked for my number and I wrote it down for him. Even though he didn't cheer for me in the fashion parade, I kindly forgave him and gave him a second chance.

When I got back from my three months in Melbourne, we went on our first real date. I still wasn't coping so well with the end of my last relationship: I felt that I was still in love with my ex-boyfriend even though I didn't want to be — I knew he was an asshole, but I couldn't move past this feeling. So I was still hitting the town, big time. Why I thought alcohol would make me feel better, I have no idea — it is a notorious depressant, after all. The night before our date, I'd been out on an all-nighter, drinking with friends and letting my emotions out as usual. So I wasn't in a good way and I came pretty close to cancelling on Mat.

I often think how different my life would have been had I not gone out with him that night. Later on, Mat confided that he wouldn't have called back if I had cancelled. I'd mucked him about a few times and he figured this would be my last chance.

Our date was on a Saturday night, and Mat came to pick me up from my place in Bronte. My garden apartment was one of four in a beautiful old Art Deco building on Palmerston Avenue, a walk away from Bronte Beach. Not long before I had also bought one of the upstairs apartments as an investment with my ex-boyfriend. His brother was living in it at the time. That evening I was careful to sneak out without him seeing me.

It was always important to me to be self-sufficient. It went against every fibre of my being to rely on a man for my finances. That's why I learnt everything I could about money from an early age, investing and strategising so I wouldn't need to be looked after. I never wanted to feel vulnerable in that sense. I worked very hard to get to the stage where I could support a family on my own if necessary; I still pride myself on being able to do that to this day, even though I don't need to right now.

Mat knocked on my front door, dead on time. I was dressed in ripped jeans, a custom-torn Bonds T-shirt covered in safety pins, chain belts and high heels. I looked as though I was going out clubbing. Mat was dressed smartly in a collared shirt, designer jeans and dress shoes. I remember his shoes clicking on the footpath as we walked out to his car.

I had always been attracted to bad boys who wore sneakers and low-slung jeans that showed their underwear. And I liked it if they could dance — that was important. But this checklist had never brought me happiness before, so maybe it was time for a change.

I had only ever had one other boyfriend who wore dress shoes on a date, and that was Lachlan Murdoch. Mat didn't remind me of him particularly, but to me dress shoes spelled maturity and sophistication, and I figured he'd treat me better than most men I had gone out with.

So off we went on our first date, him in his dress shoes and me in my bondage wear. We looked a very unlikely couple. Mat took me to an expensive Japanese restaurant that had just opened in Bondi. Clearly he thought I had class and he treated me accordingly. But as the night progressed he was reminded that I could let my hair down with the best of them.

We drank cocktails, we laughed, and we enjoyed each other's company. Then he took me home. He kissed me on the cheek — and that was it.

A few weeks out from *The X Factor* making its debut on national TV, we travelled around the country searching out the nation's talent. There was some real talent out there and we found some amazing performers. Only thing was, to find the gold we had to sift through all the freaks and losers.

Some people's parents are way too kind in encouraging them in their pursuit of stardom. Or cruel, depending on how you look at it. There was certainly an element of cruelty on *The X Factor*, and I was head of that department. My job went like this: Step 1. Identify the freaks and losers. Step 2. Get them to demonstrate their freak/loser qualities in front of the cameras. Step 3. Make them cry about how all their hopes and dreams have been shattered by the judges saying 'no'.

Soul-destroying? You bet, for them and for me. I felt that I was exploiting people whose aspirations were being crushed purely for the audience's entertainment.

At the same time I was dealing with my own demons. I knew this moment was huge for me but I just wasn't coping with the pressure of it all. Over those months on *The X Factor* I was a train wreck, pure and simple.

More and more I began turning to alcohol. I wasn't an alcoholic, but I was drinking increasing amounts to bolster my confidence. The problem was, I wasn't just drinking in social situations any more: I was drinking on the job as well. It started out as having one just before going on air, to give me enough Dutch courage to make it through. That progressed to needing a bottle of champagne on hand at all times. My producer would keep it hidden for me somewhere so I could pop off to the bathroom for a cigarette and a drink when I needed it. In the media world, live television is one of the most nerve-racking things you can do. My way of coping with it was to apply my alcohol Band-Aid in commercial breaks.

No surprise, really, that I wasn't performing at my best: lack of confidence, emotional turmoil and a magically refilling glass was a lethal mix for me. The worse I felt the more I drank, the more I drank the worse I felt. I was caught in a downward spiral. Sometimes I felt a part of me standing back and watching it happen, a car accident in slow motion.

Before and after every show, Mat would call me to tell me how awesome he thought I was, even if I clearly hadn't performed well. He was making me nervous: just a little too perfect for my liking. None of my previous boyfriends had been anywhere near as supportive. Even my parents took my appearances in their stride, after years of seeing me on-screen in various roles. I was doing a lot of different things, so I can see it was hard for them to keep up, let alone get excited. At one stage just before taking on *The X Factor* I was designing jeans and acting as an ambassador for jeans company Jeanswest, writing a column for the local paper, travelling to Africa for World Vision and working for Channel V — all at the same time.

I was still managing to hold it all together, but I could feel my fingers slipping a little.

One day when I was back in Sydney, Mat rang. 'Hey, kitten, what're you doing?'

'Not much, sugar, what's happening with you?' We'd started on the nicknames already, even though we hadn't even kissed. We talked a lot on the phone and we'd had quite a few dates by this stage, but we were taking it excruciatingly slowly. Both of us were lugging too much baggage to move any faster.

'I have to go see the doc about my heel and I've got no one to watch the kids,' Mat said. 'I can't get hold of their mum — I'll have to take them with me to the hospital.' I could hear the desperation in his voice.

'Sounds like you're in a bit of a quandary, sugar,' I said in a teasing tone. 'I'll look after them for you.'

'Really?' He sounded quite shocked.

'Why not?' I replied, suddenly unsure. What had I done? This was a big deal. Those kids were everything to him.

'OK — see you soon then,' he said. There was no mistaking the joy in his voice.

As I hung up the phone, I decided not to tell the kids that

I might be falling in love with their dad. I'd be super-nanny Chloe, just a friend who had come to babysit.

Mat's apartment in Darling Harbour was right on the water. Great views but no furniture, not even a bed: he slept on a giant beanbag-type thing called a 'Love Sac'. The first time I came over, Wallabies player Lote Tuqiri was perched inside the thing playing Mat's Playstation. That's pretty much all you could do at his place. His sole possessions were a flat-screen TV, a Playstation and the Love Sac.

I knocked on Mat's door, not knowing what to expect. Mat's nine-year-old son Jack opened it. Mat had spoken at length about his two children and we had pored over photos of them together. I had often heard him talk with them on the phone and I just loved the tone his voice took when he spoke to his kids.

'Hello, you must be Jack,' I said.

'Hi,' Jack said shyly. Then over his shoulder, he called, 'Dad, the babysitter's here!' I choked back a burst of hysterical laughter.

'Hi, babysitter,' Mat came over, smiling with his trademark sexy smirk.

'Um, hi,' I laughed nervously.

'This is Chloe, kids — Chloe, this is Jack and Skyla,' Mat said.

Jack had beautiful green eyes just like his dad, sandy blond hair and a Cronulla-boy tan. Skyla had crystal blue eyes with long dark hair, cute freckles and sticky-out ears. They were two of the most gorgeous creatures I had ever seen.

Skyla came running up and gave me a big hug. 'We're going for a swim, wanna come?' she asked me, clutching my hand.

'She loves me already!' I thought, silently humming with pride.

'I didn't bring a cozzie but I'll come and watch,' I said as she dragged me through the door.

We went up to the hotel pool, which had a spectacular view across Darling Harbour. Mat had time before his appointment, so he jumped in the pool with the kids. I watched him play in the water with them for about fifteen minutes. He would swim underwater, pick them up and throw them across the pool. Skyla would jump on his back and he would chase Jack, pretending to be a sea monster. He showered them in kisses and smothered them in cuddles. After those fifteen minutes, I had fallen head over heels for this man.

He was so loving and gentle with them both, yet playful and funny too. I could see Mat was an incredible dad to those kids and I could see how much they meant to him. He reminded me of what our dad had been like with us.

After Mat left for his appointment, I bathed the kids and got them ready for bed. We were sitting down in the Love Sac to watch some TV when Jack said, 'You look like that girl off *The X Factor.*'

'Ah, that would be because I am that girl,' I replied, laughing.

'Wow, Dad must be paying you heaps to babysit us,' he said in wonderment. Jack spent the rest of the evening trying to get out of me just how much his dad was coughing up for this honour.

5

Yet always when I look death in the face,
When I clamber to the heights of sleep,
Or when I grow excited with wine,
Suddenly I meet your face.

— W.B. Yeats, 'A Deep-Sworn Vow'

The very first time I watched Mat play a game of union I really had no idea. Dad and the rest of my family were huge rugby union nuts, but I was just never interested. My weekends were about pursuing my passion for music, and sport just didn't figure. You could ask me anything about music and I would talk until the cows came home, but football was a different ball game — literally.

One weekend, Mat invited me and some of my girlfriends to the members stand at Aussie Stadium in Sydney to watch the Waratahs versus Crusaders game. I spent hours on the phone with my friends the night before, debating the crucial question: what should we wear? We finally came to the conclusion that it would be similar to the members area at the races, with which we were very familiar. We should definitely get dressed up to the nines: designer dresses, stilettos — the works.

It didn't take us long after arriving to realise that pretty much everyone else was in rugby jerseys. We looked a bit ridiculous. Hot, but ridiculous.

When the team ran out onto the field, people cheered loudly for their favourite players. Mat got a massive cheer.

'Shit, he must be pretty good!' I turned to my girlfriends, but they were too busy checking out the talent in the stands to pay attention to what was happening on the field.

As Mat ran out, he turned around and looked up at the stand. Spotting me, he waved. My heart skipped a beat.

While most of my girlfriends (except Tara, who was quite the rugby buff) talent-spotted, the two of us really got into watching the game. Mat ended up scoring a try and being awarded Man of the Match. Afterwards I said to him, 'Wow, you played really well. And you scored a goal thingy — congratulations!'

'A try,' he corrected me gently.

'Yes, you tried really hard and you got it — good work!' I said. I had so much to learn.

As our relationship deepened, I was travelling regularly between Sydney and Melbourne, filming the live shows of *The X Factor* and *The Xtra Factor*. All the travel was putting a strain on the relationship — well, that and the fact that I was becoming a little too fond of alcohol as a way of dispelling the stress and anxiety of being on live national TV.

For the very first live show I had no autocue, so they had decided to write my script on pieces of cardboard. I don't use autocue or dummy cards as a rule, never had in four years of live television. I did, however, want to keep this job, so I just went along with what I was told to do. As usual, I had a bottle of something nearby to keep my courage up. It was a complete disaster: the guy holding the cards got them mixed up and I was all over the shop.

Mat was touring South Africa with the Wallabies that year, but because of my TV and media commitments I couldn't go with him. The night before he left, I finally spent the night at his place. It was made easier — or more comfortable, at least — by the fact that his hotel room now had furniture in it. We had spent a day in Freedom and Ikea picking out a few things so he could live there properly. I'm afraid the Love Sac just wasn't going to cut it.

In the morning, I drove Mat to the airport with his bags. As we pulled up at the international terminal, his teammates were arriving too, dropped off by wives and girlfriends. Stirling Mortlock gave Mat a nod as he got out of his wife's car then looked at me quizzically.

'I want you to be my girlfriend now,' Mat said rather coltishly. 'Can you be my girlfriend?'

'OK then,' I replied, and that was the beginning of a crazy relationship. Crazy because we were both spinning out of control. Together, we were in the habit of wanting to party all the time, and it wasn't healthy. When the kids were around we held it together for their sake, but we had a lot to get out of our systems. Both of us had a lot of baggage; our theme song was Erykah Badu's 'Bag Lady'. Seeing her live in concert many years later, I wept, remembering all of the baggage we had been carrying and had finally left behind.

After a couple of months of phone calls and dates, Mat called me late one night. He had taken a sleeping tablet, which he often did after he was injured or played a tough game. He never went straight to bed after he took them, opting instead to fight it and stay awake so that he could wind down from the adrenalin rush of the game. I had had my usual bottle of wine to put myself to sleep. What ensued neither of us can really recall, but the upshot was that it was over. We had broken up.

As our relationship was hitting the skids, so too were the ratings for *The X Factor*. *Australian Idol* had just finished, *American Idol* had just started, *Pop Stars* had kicked off on Channel 7 — there were simply too many reality talent shows.

Eventually the series ended without too much fanfare. The winners were a group of five boys called 'Random', who were absolutely brilliant. But we knew that was it: we didn't expect there would be another season of the show.

Blogs and discussion boards were packed with people saying how much they disliked me and what a ditz I was. I needed a change of scenery. My sister Camilla had just moved to America. She was a talented actor with a passion for theatre, and she had scored a scholarship to train at the American Academy of Dramatic Arts in New York City — the same place Lauren

Bacall, Robert Redford and Kirk Douglas trained, to name but a few. I decided to go and visit her — much to her dismay, as I wasn't particularly interested in sightseeing, just in drinking my sorrow away. That I did and then some. I only remember snippets of my whirlwind tour of the States: some time in Hawaii, San Francisco, then annoying my sister in New York.

I had to come back to reality eventually, and when I did I decided it was time to get rid of a few bad memories. My apartment had to go, for starters: I'd lived in that place for almost ten years and there were too many ghosts for me to move forward while I lived there. So as soon as I got back from the States I put it on the market. I put all my furniture in storage, got in an interior decorator to style the apartment so it looked perfect, then I moved out.

At twenty-eight with two cats in tow, I moved back in with my mum. She was happy to have us, but I wasn't too impressed. No house, no partner, almost thirty and living with my mum — awesome!

Mum was pretty good to me, though. She really tried to cheer me up. My birthday was coming up and I was organising a dinner with a few close friends at a Japanese restaurant in Surry Hills. When I got off the phone to a friend one night, out of the blue my mum said, 'Why don't you call Mat and invite him to your birthday dinner?' We were sitting in the backyard drinking wine and smoking cigarettes, as was our nightly tradition.

'I really liked Mat,' she said, lighting another cigarette off the butt of her previous one. 'And so did your grandma.'

She was right. All my family had loved him, which was really rare for a boyfriend of mine. He had been a real gentleman, and I missed his gorgeous kids just as much as I missed him. All of a sudden I knew that I wanted to be with him more than ever before.

'Alright, I will,' I said. I picked up the phone and pressed the button next to his name. It started ringing and I held my breath.

'Hello,' came his husky voice down the line. I could tell he was smiling.

'Um — hi, remember me?' I said in a weak attempt at humour.

And so we began our relationship again, but this time we were ready for each other.

Mat and I lived together briefly at his apartment in Darling Harbour until we decided to move to Cronulla to be closer to the kids. They had been staying with us regularly and it was proving too taxing to get them to school in Cronulla, thirty kilometres away, on time. So we made the move to the Shire, or 'God's country' as the residents call it.

We moved into a beautiful old house at Gunnamatta Bay. With three bedrooms and two bathrooms, there was just enough space for all of us. Best of all there was a playroom downstairs and a path that led to a private beach. I really loved it, but it was a little far for my close girlfriends to travel. I began seeing less and less of them, much to my dismay.

Our relationship became quite serious quite quickly, and we began talking babies. I had always wanted to have children. Ever since I was a little girl I dreamed about what my kids would be like: what they would look like, their personalities, how I would nurture them and the values I would instil in them. I respected Mat so much because he was prepared to go through it all again and have more kids for me. I quickly discovered, though, that he wasn't just doing it for me — he absolutely adores kids. Even now we would have more if it weren't for me putting my foot down. So although we hadn't planned to get pregnant, we both said that if it happened we would be over the moon.

I was still doing bits and pieces of work, nothing big, until one day I got a call from my agent. Ursula was my mentor and the one who had discovered me all those years ago. Ursula Hufnagl had been a famous model in her day and now she ran Chic Management model agency in Sydney, which looks after some of the biggest models in the world as well as a lot of high-profile media stars. They are the best at what they do. She was also like a surrogate mother to me — I even called her 'Mum'. I love and respect her so much: she had always cared so much about my career that I knew she would never let me put a foot wrong, professionally.

'It appears they really want you for this movie,' Ursula told me.

'What do you think, Mum?' I always asked for her opinion on everything workwise.

'I think it could be great for you to brush up on your skills again,' Ursula replied.

'OK, I'll do it,' I said, excited and very upbeat.

I hadn't done a movie since *Under the Radar*, a comedy/thriller that came out in 2004. I really didn't consider myself to have any acting ability — not like my sister Camilla, anyway. Some of the behind-the-scenes crew had the same opinion: one of the audio guys made me cry with his scathing comments. 'Now we've got the real acting out of the way,' he would jibe when I walked on set to shoot a scene. No one expected much of me, so when I was nominated for an AFI (Australian Film Institute) award for my role as Jo the triumph was extra sweet.

This new film was a low budget production, but that didn't bother me. I had so much fun making movies because I really enjoyed the creative process. It was to be shot in January 2006, so Mat and I decided we should wait until after that to consider trying for a child.

For some time, I had been complaining to Mat about pains in my side. This constant dull ache made me fear the worst and I was worried that there was something terribly wrong with me. 'I think I might have a cyst or something,' I said to Mat one day. So off to the doctor I went. Among other things he did a pregnancy test and that was it — I was pregnant.

So that's how we found out we had conceived Max. The movie I was all set to do never eventuated: not only was it low budget, it was hit with budget problems, so it never came to be. The path was clear and I knew we were meant to have this baby.

* * *

As a professional rugby player, Mat would travel overseas for long periods of time. These guys spent six months of the year abroad, away from their families and the people they loved. They were paid very well, but their personal lives took a beating.

Long before I knew I was pregnant I decided to travel to Europe to meet up with Mat while he was playing for the Wallabies. One of my best friends, Tara (the rugby buff), was living in Barcelona so I flew to Spain to visit her with my good friend Adrian, who travelled with me to the States when Mat and I broke up. Now I would be travelling in the first stages of pregnancy, and it was going to be really hard to keep that a secret from two of my close friends. I wouldn't be drinking for a start, which for me was extremely suspicious.

When we had checked in at the airport, Adrian made his usual suggestion. 'Let's go get a beer.'

'Um — sure,' I said, realising he would need to be sitting down with a beer in his hand when I hit him with this particular news.

'What do you want, a Corona?' Adrian asked, gesturing to the bartender in the airport lounge.

'I'm good, actually. Maybe just a soda water.' All of a sudden it was as if time stood still. The whole bar seemed to go silent as Adrian slowly turned his head toward me.

'Soda water!' he looked angrily at me for a minute. Then he threw his head back and laughed wildly.

'Good one, yeah. Two Coronas, thanks,' he waved his cash at the bartender.

'I'm pregnant, Adrian,' I blurted out.

'Make that one Corona!' he shouted across the bar. 'Are you kidding me?' he asked, waiting for me to start laughing.

'No, I'm actually about four weeks pregnant,' I said, tapping my belly absently.

'OK. Sorry, two Coronas, thanks,' he gestured back at the bartender, who seemed unsure whether he was coming or going at this stage. When the beers arrived Adrian sculled one and then the other.

'Congratulations!' He gave me a big squeeze. 'That's awesome, Chloe, I'm really happy for you.'

Barcelona was amazing. It was my third time there, but this time there was no sangria and plenty more sightseeing. Most mornings I woke up and went for a jog while it was still dark outside. Mat, Tara and Adrian had always partied the night before, so they were never up at daybreak. Alone I explored that beautiful city in the newborn light of morning, and thought constantly about the little person who was miraculously growing inside me.

'One day we will come back here together,' I would whisper to my tummy. I wanted my baby to see La Sagrada Família, the stunning cathedral designed by Gaudí and still under construction today, long after his death. I dreamed of one day taking my child through the many halls of the Picasso Museum and eating paella together under the setting Spanish sun.

6

The blood-dimmed tide is loosed, and everywhere
The ceremony of innocence is drowned …

— W.B. Yeats, 'The Second Coming'

3 January 2006, 8 a.m.: I wake to the familiar sound of a text message coming through on my phone. Reaching over, it felt as if my tummy had grown during the night. Was that possible? As I grabbed the phone and fumbled with the keys, even my fingers felt fatter. I'd read about swollen ankles during pregnancy, but fingers?

The text was from our neighbour, Martin Downs, asking Mat to call him as soon as possible. Right now, Mat was sleeping. We had only just got back from Byron Bay, where we'd spent New Year's Eve with some of my friends. For the life of me I couldn't remember spending a New Year sober before — not since I was a kid, anyway. It was hilarious, watching people get more and more intoxicated and talking absolute rubbish.

Looking again at my phone, I considered how unusual it was for me to be still in bed at this time. I was three months pregnant, and while I was pregnant I got up around five to go for a walk most mornings. I relished that time, thinking about the little person I was making inside of me. That was our special time: my baby's and mine.

I got up and put on clothes to go walking. Gunnamatta Bay was a beautiful area to walk in: I would go down onto our private beach, walk past the sheltered bay and the mansions flanking it, then through parklands and up to the oval. It was particularly quiet that morning: being school holidays and early in the new year, not many people were about. Walking later than usual, I began to feel the heat of the sun more intensely. I noticed on my phone that there were more missed text messages and phone calls from Martin — or Downsy, as we called him. I must have knocked the phone onto silent. I decided to give him a call to see what the fuss was about.

Downsy was a retired undercover cop who lived next door to us with his wife and six kids. Coincidentally, as well as being our neighbour he had been a good friend of Mat's dad Steve — or Sludge, as all his closest friends called him — for many years. Downsy was a colourful character who seemed to know everyone, and an incurable joker: he was always playing tricks on people and there was never a dull moment when he was around. But when he answered his phone this particular morning, his tone was more serious than I had ever heard it.

'I need to speak to Mat right away,' he said. 'People have been trying to contact him all morning, Chloe — his phone must be off.'

'What's wrong? What's happened, Downsy?' I asked.

'It's Sludge. Chloe, something's happened to Steve.' The minute I heard Downsy use Steve's proper name, I knew something was terribly wrong.

We had had dinner with Steve a few weeks earlier. Just before Christmas we told him the news about our baby, and he was over the moon for us.

The family had come through a difficult few years: Mat's mother Carol had died five years before after a long and excruciating battle with breast cancer, so good news was particularly precious. Steve and his second wife Ingrid had been travelling overseas through the holidays and hadn't long been back. It appeared, in fact, that Steve had come back without Ingrid. According to Mat, they had had a falling out. While we were in Byron Bay Mat had a message on his phone from his dad, asking him to call. We had been in and out of range, so Mat hadn't rung back yet. I suddenly felt sick to my stomach.

'We need to get Mat over to his dad's right away. I think he's dead, Chloe! Tell Mat I'm coming to get him now. Don't tell him anything yet, just tell him I'm coming to get him. Oh my God, I'm so sorry ...'

I hung up the phone in shock. 'God, this can't be happening,' I thought.

Jack and Skyla were still asleep when I got back to the house. We had picked them up from their mum's house when we got back from our holiday and they were so happy to see their dad. They adored him. They adored their 'Poppy', Steve, too.

I didn't think I could cope with this emotional burden. 'What should I do?' I asked no one in particular.

I decided not to alarm Mat or the children. I'm no drama queen anyway, and I didn't want to over-dramatise this situation: maybe Downsy was overreacting, as he was known to do.

Mat was still sleeping. 'Darling, wake up.' I shook him lightly. 'Darling, it's your dad — you have to get over to his place right away.'

'What?' he rolled out of bed, still half asleep.

'Just get in the shower, Downsy will drive you over,' I said, pulling some clothes out of his drawers for him. He was still too asleep to argue with me.

As soon as the shower stopped, the front door bell rang. It was Downsy.

'He's just getting out of the shower,' I told Downsy. I stood there staring at him as he leaned against the doorframe, his face white and fallen. He was simply shaking his head in disbelief. I didn't dare speak in case the words brought something dreadful into existence. I just hoped there was a mistake and they would come back laughing and joking as they usually did.

Mat gave me a kiss and greeted Downsy at the door. 'What's happening?' he asked in his usual upbeat, comical way.

'We'll talk in the car,' Downsy replied in a monotone. Mat

looked back at me with a strained, bemused smile. Downsy looked at me gravely then pulled the door shut behind them.

'Shit!' I exclaimed under my breath.

As soon as they had gone I rang Michelle, Jack and Skyla's mum. No answer. I left a message. 'Michelle, it's Chloe here. I was hoping I could drop the kids with you. Something has happened to Steve ...' my voice faltered. 'Please call me.'

Michelle called back eventually and said it was OK to drop Jack and Skyla with her. After taking them to her house, I drove on to Sludge's place. Outside the apartment block, there were press and police and people everywhere.

Downsy was standing there as I pulled up. 'What's happening?' I asked, dreading the answer.

'Mat's gone inside to identify the body. He hasn't come out yet,' Downsy said. I could tell he had been crying.

'The ambulance is on its way but I think it's a bit late,' Martin said as we both stared at the entrance to the building. Tears stung my cheeks.

'I was just walking past when I saw something going on outside Steve's place. Ingrid's brother went to check on Sludge and he found him. Apparently Ingrid was worried he wasn't answering her calls so she asked her brother to go over. He just lives around the ...' his voice trailed off.

A figure had appeared in the doorway of the building. It was Mat. He stumbled out into the sunlight and wailed aloud in pain as everyone looked on in horror.

I ran to comfort him. Mat's knees buckled as he took in the fact that his dad was gone; his hero was no longer. For a moment I was supporting my unborn baby as well as his father: my love for them both gave me a strength I didn't know I possessed.

'It's Dad! He's gone! He was just lying there like he was asleep …' Mat sobbed, his face contorting with pain.

I helped him to sit down on the step as his body began to convulse with heart-wrenching sobs. He was holding a gold watch in his hand, rubbing it over and over with his thumb and staring at it through his tears.

For some time, I couldn't bring myself to speak. I merely sat there, trying to absorb some of the pain the father of my child must be feeling at that moment.

I have never seen a man so grief-stricken. My heart was breaking for him. Mat glanced at my pregnant belly then stood up again and collapsed in my arms, overwhelmed with grief.

The watch was Steve's Tag Heuer. Mat must have slipped it off his wrist while he knelt beside him in the stairway. It was something tangible to hold onto, something personal of his dad's that he still wears, years later.

'The police said he left notes for me, Don, Mel and Ingrid,' Mat said as we walked slowly back to the car. 'They'll give them to us when they finish studying them.'

'Oh no,' I said, absorbing the significance of this piece of information.

'The police also said that he might have tried to dial triple zero before he died,' his voice trailed off.

Mat's phone began ringing the minute he got back in the car. 'Who is it?' I asked as we pulled away from his dad's building.

'Blocked number,' Mat said flatly. 'Probably a journo wanting a quote.' As he looked out the window, I could see his reflection; tears were still streaming down his face.

Mat was well used to the guerrilla tactics of the press. He had experienced it many times before because of his 'bad boy' behaviour, both on and off the field. They were relentless, and this time heartless too. The vision of his father slumped dead in a stairwell was still fresh in his mind, yet the reporters had to have a quote to sell some more papers.

By the time we got home, Mat's phone was ringing again. Mat opened the door of my little white Mercedes but that was as far as he got. He seemed to be in a daze, his face red and still wet with tears. He looked absently at his phone.

'Blocked number,' he mumbled as I helped him out of the car. When he stood up he passed the phone to me. 'I can't do this. Can you take it?' His voice was quivering with emotion.

I reached out and grabbed the phone. In that moment, I went into defence mode. Putting my hands on his shoulders and looking into his bloodshot eyes, I said, 'I am going to take care of you and all of this.'

As Mat embraced me I felt his body shake, and tears welled in my tired eyes. 'I love you,' I said.

'I love you too. So much,' he replied.

We walked slowly into the house, Mat clutching me for support. Mat went to the fridge and opened a beer then stepped out onto the balcony. Overlooking Gunnamatta Bay and the beach below, it made a serene setting for melancholy thoughts. He took a sip of beer and let his head fall into his hands.

I went to the bathroom — something you do a lot of when you're pregnant. As soon as I shut the door, my strong exterior crumbled. I sat on the toilet and bawled my eyes out in absolute silence so Mat wouldn't hear me. I had to be strong for him; he needed me to be that right now. I resolved that this would not break us, and I believed it would all depend on the strength in me. Mat's strength — mental and physical — was something I had always been in awe of. I felt safe with him, as though nothing and no one could hurt me. Now I had to be the strong one, or at least try to be. I hauled myself up and rinsed my face under the tap. The cold water felt fresh and real.

Suddenly I heard voices outside. I opened the door to find a cluster of Mat's relatives standing on the step with cases of beer and bottles of wine in their hands and devastation written across their faces.

One by one I hugged them as they filed in and gathered around Mat on the balcony. 'More strength,' I whispered, grateful for the company.

As I turned to shut the door I noticed some cameras and a television truck across the road. I slammed the door quickly and went inside. 'There's press camped out across the street, darling,' I said softly to Mat. He seemed to be in a trance as his family buzzed around him. Lost in thoughts of his dad perhaps, trying to lock those memories in his mind now that they were all he had left.

'I'm going to have to hold a press conference,' Mat said suddenly, breaking out of his trance-like state. Everyone around him went quiet.

'They'll keep bothering us until we give them something,' Mat's brother Don agreed.

So it was decided. Mat began making arrangements through his media contacts. The conference would be held at the Sharks Rugby League Club the next day. Slowly, Mat's family and friends filtered off home towards the end of the day and we began preparing for the press conference.

We woke up the next morning in a daze, with a surreal sense of yesterday's events hanging over us. Mat was up early and on the balcony when I got out of bed. He had a pen and paper in front of him and a cup of tea in his hand. Hearing me come down the creaky stairs, he looked up at me. His eyes were still bloodshot and he looked very tired — I doubt that he had slept a wink. He managed a weak smile as I kissed him on the head and sat down opposite him.

'Working on something to say at the press conference,' he said, refocusing on the paper in front of him. I looked out at a ferry making its way across the bay. Today was going to be difficult.

'You don't want me to come with you, do you?' I asked, not knowing what his response might be.

'I don't want you to come — I *need* you to come,' he said, holding my hand across the table. 'I need you with me.'

'I'll be there,' I said, leaning over and kissing him lightly on the lips.

The amount of media interest in Steve's passing astonished me. I knew he was a football great but I had no idea just how great. He was a hero, particularly in his home town. When we arrived at the club for the press conference, we saw countless television trucks and paparazzi in the car park. Once they realised who was in our car they began snapping away.

As we walked together from the car to the entrance, Mat held my hand so firmly it almost hurt. I squeezed his hand back to let him know I wasn't going anywhere.

Inside, Mat and his brother Don were ushered to the front of the room. I kissed Mat his brother and squeezed his hand, then hung back on the outskirts of the throng. Looking around the mass of reporters from the top radio stations, newspapers and television networks, I felt that they were ravenous for whatever words Mat might throw their way. This was a big story and no one had a quote from the football star's famous son yet. Mat and Don reached the podium and Don patted his brother affectionately on the back as they sat down side by side.

Mat had not yet looked up at the crowd in front of him, but the camera flashes highlighted the tears glistening on his cheeks. He pulled out the paper he had been scribbling on earlier that morning. As he unfolded it slowly I could see his hands were shaking.

'Dad's sudden, unexpected death has been a tremendous shock to all of us.' Mat's green eyes glanced up from the paper briefly as the cameras flashed. 'He was suffering from some depression and, as a person of his stature and a public figure, he found it really hard to talk about it to other people and therefore exacerbated the problem.' His voice faltered a little.

Barry Pierce, the Cronulla Club president, said a few words when Mat had finished. 'There will be no questions and the family have asked that the media please respect their privacy.' This was met with an agitated hum from the journalists. Clearly they were not satisfied with that statement. There was obviously not enough dirt for them to help sell their papers. But the question of just how exactly Steve Rogers died would be answered by the coroner, so they would have to wait.

Waiting, however, does not sell papers, so a few journalists approached the family for quotes. One paper even sent a reporter down to the local pub and plied some of Steve's relatives with booze to get some controversial snippets. These techniques got them quotes ranging from, 'Steve was an alcoholic,' to, 'Steve had a very bad gambling problem.' Why Steve's mates and relatives thought it was a good idea to say these things was absolutely beyond me.

Mat was furious. He had told the family to keep quiet until they knew exactly what had happened, but some people wanted their five minutes of fame, a last ride on the wave of Steve's celebrity.

Meanwhile, we had a funeral to arrange. Seeing how devastated Mat was, I decided to take over all of the preparations. He hadn't long seen his mother buried, so I wanted to do anything I could to ease the pain he was feeling. We also finally received back from the police the notes Steve wrote. They appeared to be his last words to his kids. This cemented to us that he had meant to say goodbye, even though the coroner would later deem his death 'accidental'.

This funeral was going to be a major public event as well as a private farewell. Steve was an icon in the community, having captained Australia's league team and played for Cronulla for many years. We chose to hold the send-off at the Shire Christian Centre, so I set up a meeting with the pastor, Mike Murphy, to discuss the protocol.

He came to our house, which for several days had had media camped out the front, hoping to get a quote or a picture of tearful family members, despite Mat's plea to let us grieve in peace.

We had been waiting over an hour for Steve's wife Ingrid to arrive. The pastor had more than his fair share of English Breakfast tea and I was starting to feel embarrassed when she finally called.

'Hi, Chloe, how are you?' Ingrid said in a surprisingly upbeat tone.

'Good thanks, Ingrid — how far away are you?' I asked, trying not to sound annoyed.

'Just around the corner — sorry, I was getting my hair done. Are there any paparazzi out the front?'

'No, I don't think so,' I replied, looking out the front door.

'Oh. OK, we'll be there soon,' she replied. Ten minutes later she finally arrived, looking very glamorous for our meeting with the pastor. I introduced her to Pastor Mike and we set about talking through the logistics of what would be no ordinary funeral for no ordinary man.

The funeral parlour had suggested that close family members come to view the body and say their last goodbyes. I remember standing in the sun in front of the building, watching Don and his girlfriend Danny smoke cigarettes, with Mat's sister Melanie and her husband Shane standing by while we waited for Ingrid to arrive. Her tardiness was beginning to get on Mat's nerves. I understand that everyone deals with grief in a different way but the rest of the family was having to wait for Ingrid a little too much. After half an hour, Mat made a decision.

'We're going in. I'm not waiting for her any longer.' Mat pushed open the door and walked through to reception. The lady at the desk recognised us straight away; I vaguely remembered speaking to her when we came in a few days earlier to choose the coffin and floral arrangements.

'Come right this way, Mr Rogers,' she said, acknowledging the rest of us with a smile and a nod. We walked through and came to a door. It was your average door, very plain, no elaborate sign saying 'Ashes to ashes' or anything like that.

'Steve's behind this door right now,' she said. Tears began to form in our eyes. For a moment, it sounded as though Steve was alive and when she opened the door he might yell, 'Surprise!' then hug and kiss his boys as he always did.

Steve had adored his boys. He didn't always show it: he was a tough man, judging from the stories Mat told and the short time I had known him. But every time he greeted his sons you could see a flicker of pride as he kissed them unabashedly. I hadn't known many men to greet their grown sons with a kiss.

'Will all of you be staying to view?' she gestured at Danny and me and Mel's husband Shane.

'Do you want us to stay?' I asked Mat, not sure if this was something I should be part of.

'I need you here,' he replied, squeezing my hand.

I felt a shiver run down my spine as we walked through and saw the coffin. Danny, Shane and I stood at the back of the room as Mat, Melanie and Don walked up to the coffin side by side. They looked down at their dad, touched his cold hands and embraced him, leaning over the coffin and sobbing in immeasurable pain.

'Why, Dad, why did you have to leave us?' Mat cried, leaning down to kiss his dad on the forehead for the last time. His tears spilled onto his father's cheeks, until it looked as though Steve was crying too.

I couldn't hold back the tears; my pregnant body shook all over. I wanted to comfort Mat but I had nothing to offer him that would take that pain away. Such pain, losing your dad so early in life — Steve was only fifty-one when he died. And just a few years earlier these three had lost their mum too. So much pain in such a short time.

We spent half an hour or so with Steve, then Mat, Don and Melanie finally decided it was time to go. Mat walked over to me and we embraced. I kissed his wet cheek and stroked his hair as he leaned on my shoulder.

'Let's go,' he said, lifting his head.

We made our way back through the door and out into the street. It was brighter outside than I remembered it had been when we arrived. Ingrid and some of her family were just walking in as we were leaving.

'Hello,' she said brightly. None of us were in any mood to chat, so we continued on to the car.

I had never seen a dead body before. I was trying to remain strong for Mat but inside I was shattered.

On the day of the funeral, chaos ruled at our house. I was almost four months pregnant with Max; Mat's sister Melanie was staying with us, together with her husband Shane. They had flown across from Perth a few days earlier to be there for Steve's funeral. Throughout the morning other friends and relatives came and went as I kept busy helping everyone get ready.

The day before I had gone to the church to drop off a few things. I had asked Ingrid to give me the best photo she had of Steve, which I had blown up and framed to put on his coffin. As I hurried along the footpath to the church I saw a news crew shooting out front. I dashed inside, hoping they hadn't seen me. Since the press conference, Mat and I had been trying to avoid any media. There really was nothing more to say. Unfortunately, the suspicious circumstances of Steve's death left many questions unanswered and the press were having a field day.

Mat, Don and I stayed up late that night downloading Steve's favourite songs and reminiscing. We chose various songs for the funeral, making up CDs for arrival, departure and for the wake. I felt very honoured to be part of this special time for Steve's three children. There were plenty of happy memories but some dark ones, too. I was slowly becoming aware of just how many skeletons and secrets the family had. Mat's mother was one of thirteen kids. There were two different fathers, a lot of hardship and some abuse. Mat's aunt Wendy McGregor wrote a book about that side of the family called *Oh My God!*, which about sums it up. To this day, Mat refuses to read it.

A great friend of Steve's, Craig 'Cliffo' Clifton, had put together a tribute DVD using archive footage from Channel Nine, showing Steve's successes as a Cronulla Shark and captain of the Kangaroos, Australia's national rugby league team. It was to be played at the service, so when he dropped it off the night before, we sat down to watch it. Steve had retired as a footballer by the time I met him and since I had never followed league before I met Mat, I had never seen him play. I was gobsmacked by the talent he so obviously possessed on the football field. The tribute was set to the Police song 'Walking on the Moon'; it was completely fitting because in slow motion, many of his tries were just unbelievable. Don, Mel, Mat and I sobbed uncontrollably as we watched Steve accepting his Dally M (rugby league's most prestigious prize) in 1981 with their mother Carol at his side.

When it came time to leave for the church, Don presented Mat with some cufflinks bearing the initials SR. Don had had a set made for each of them. Sitting in the lounge while Mel blow-dried my hair for me, I looked up to see two figures standing in the hallway. Don and Mat were silently helping each other put the symbolic cufflinks on. Both men's hands were far from steady, but once the cufflinks were in place the brothers embraced, burying their faces in each other's shoulders. They stood there like that for several minutes, silent but shaking with sobs. My heart broke for them.

We rely on our parents to be there always, to help us pick up the inevitable pieces or to offer that unconditional love and support you can't get anywhere else. I often took it for granted, but it was something Mat would gently remind me of over the years whenever I had disagreements with my mum or dad. 'At least you still have parents, darling. Be grateful.' His words never failed to prompt me to right any wrongs with them. I was grateful for my parents; I was also incredibly grateful for him.

Craig Pinn, a great friend of Steve's and his family, drove us to the funeral. As we turned the corner into the street where the church was, we saw it was lined with people. Hundreds of thousands of men, women and children had turned up to honour a Cronulla legend. It was overwhelming.

Strangers called out condolences and reached out to shake hands with the boys as we proceeded up the steps of the church. Inside, Mat, Mel and Don walked to the front of the church together, their gazes fixed on the coffin with the photo of Steve placed on top.

There was not a dry eye in the place through the service. Mat got up and spoke beautifully about the great memories he had of his father. Don sang an acoustic version of 'Yes I Will', a Michael Franti & Spearhead song. Melanie was the last of Steve's three children to speak. She spoke of seeing a white butterfly just that morning, and how it lifted her spirits as it reminded her that when they said their goodbyes to their mother, they had set free hundreds of white butterflies. Mel believed this was a sign that their mother was with them on this day, reassuring them that she would take good care of Steve in heaven. They were together now.

7

All things fall and are built again …

— W.B. Yeats, 'Lapis Lazuli'

After the funeral, the press was still stalking the family, trying to sniff out any controversy they could in lieu of the coroner's report. It made sense to get away until the fuss died down so Mat and I, together with Don and his girlfriend Danny, decided to take off to Lord Howe Island.

I had never been to Lord Howe Island before, but Mat and Don had fond memories of time spent there as children with their mum and dad. Mat's dad had had a great friend there who worked on a fishing tour boat, 'Crom'. He had offered to look after us while we were there.

Mat had taken time off from training with the Waratahs. The coach, Ewen McKenzie, told him to take as long as he needed to get his head straight. So the day after the funeral the four of us headed off.

The airport was reasonably busy that day, filled with people in a hurry. I had spent a lot of time in airports over the years, mainly for work. Sometimes people would recognise me but mostly they are too busy coming or going. This day, though, it seemed as though everyone was staring at us. We checked in, all four of us with our sunglasses on.

'Sorry to hear about your dad,' the guy behind the counter offered as he printed our boarding passes and placed them on the counter.

'Thanks,' Mat mumbled as he snatched the passes up. We hurried to join the queue to go through the security screening point. As we waited our turn for our bags to be scanned, I could see a couple of the guys working there begin to whisper to each other while looking at Mat. When we went through the x-ray machines one of them said, 'Condolences, Mat.'

I could see Mat was becoming increasingly agitated. We walked briskly to the Qantas lounge. Danny and I stopped at the newspaper stand to pick up some magazines for the flight. On prominent display was the front page of that day's newspaper, featuring a photo of Mat and I walking in to the funeral. I tried to cover it up before he saw it, but it was too late. Mat grabbed one and started flicking through it. Over his shoulder I caught a glimpse of a photo of the coffin being carried out by Mat, Donny and the other pallbearers. I looked up at Mat: beneath his sunglasses, a single tear was running down his cheek. He brushed it away before anyone else could see it, paid for the paper and clutched my hand tight while we continued on to the lounge.

It was going to be a hard and long road for Mat and Don to move on from this. Everywhere they went they would be reminded of their father's passing.

Mat and Don sat together in the lounge, reading the article in the paper. I imagined them as two little boys, huddling together for protection. They were openly weeping and they didn't care who saw. When Donny turned the page, I noticed something glinting on his finger. It was a gold ring with a shark on it — Steve's ring marking two hundred games for the Cronulla Sharks. I began to weep, and Danny started crying too.

Our time on Lord Howe Island was absolutely magical. We swam, ate good food and relished each others' company. While we were there, Don proposed to Danny. Although they didn't know at the time, they also conceived a child there — a little girl who would be called Eden.

We had gone to Lord Howe Island leaving Jack and Skyla with their mum, and we missed them terribly. On our return we took them to spend a few days at my dad's farm in Rydal, a little town just past the Blue Mountains, not far from Lithgow. My father had bought the property 'Chapel House' from the famous artist John Olsen; drenched in history, it included several buildings and the most incredible heritage-listed gardens. The dirt road leading up to the main house was lined with prunus trees and conifers, with a big pond on the right where ducks and geese floated peacefully. To reach the pond you walked through a beautiful rose garden. Dad and his second wife Jo worked their fingers to the bone in the garden every weekend to keep it up to scratch for public viewing; gardening was a favourite pastime for my dad, who inherited his green fingers from my grandmother.

I hoped that the beauty and peace of the farm would be good for Jack and Skyla. They had both been terribly affected by their 'Poppy's' passing: it was the second time they had attended a funeral in their short lives, the first being for their Nan, Mat's mum.

It was a stunningly clear night and we had just finished eating an awesome dinner of Jo's exotic salads, together with steaks that Mat helped Dad cook on his big barbecue under the stars. I loved coming out here and seeing the star-studded universe without the interruption of city smog. The world fell into perspective out here, and we were reminded that we were just specks in the grand scheme of things.

The kids had headed up to the pond to check the yabby trap Dad had helped them put in when we arrived that afternoon. Mat and I were sitting back with Dad and Jo, talking about our time on Lord Howe Island. Then the topic turned to Steve and the funeral. Dad and Jo had come along to show their support, even though they had never met Steve.

'I just can't believe he's gone.' Mat shook his head, his eyes filling with tears. 'He only texted me the day before to say he really wanted to catch up.'

I suddenly began to get emotional, watching him hurt again. I was four months pregnant by now, prone to all of the hormonal surges that come with that state as well as the events that had devastated our world this past month.

The kids had come back up from the pond; Jack had a big yabby in his hands. Dad and Mat jumped up to help him into the kitchen with it. Seeing me upset, Skyla came running over to me and squeezed me in one of her loving hugs.

'Don't be sad, Chloe,' she said.

I kissed her softly on the head. 'I'll be OK, Bub.' Everyone called her Bub, even Jack. She gave me a big kiss on the cheek and went inside to watch television with Jack.

Jo sat across the table from me with a strange look on her face.

'Why were you never like that with me?' she asked. I looked over at Dad and Mat in the kitchen, deep in conversation as they put the yabby in a pot to cook the next day.

'I don't know, Jo. But I don't think now is the time to talk about this.' I pushed my chair out from the table and began piling up the dirty plates. As I walked into the kitchen, she followed me.

'Why is now not the time?' she asked, her voice breaking with emotion.

'I'm sorry, Jo, but you can't expect to just start a relationship like that with me right now!' I was starting to get emotional again. 'You never hugged or kissed me as a child. I'm almost thirty years old, it's a bit late to have that now.' I was really beginning to want a drink, even though I'd hated the smell of wine since I became pregnant.

Dad and Mat had had their backs to us at the sink but they both turned around to us in shock. 'What's going on? Is everything OK?' Dad asked, walking over to Jo.

'You always took her side!' Jo ran out to the cottage next door with my dad close behind her. I ran outside too and, sitting on the secluded bench beside the pond, cried into the black of the night like I had never cried before. All of the pent-up emotion of the past month, plus years of family turmoil, came pouring out. I was still sitting there, howling, when Mat's arms reached around me from out of the darkness.

'What the hell is going on?' he asked, shocked by Jo's outburst and my frenzied tears.

'I don't know. Darling, I want to go home!' My sobs shook my pregnant belly to the core.

All these years later, I understand now why she exploded at me. Being a stepmother is thankless work. You try so hard to please everyone, yet no matter how much you do for your stepkids they throw it back in your face and tell you that you are not their mum. You have to deal with clashes with the children's mother, whether directly or indirectly. When the children attack the man you love and you see how much it hurts them all, there is nothing you can do but bite your tongue. I guess after sixteen years of biting her tongue, it all became too much for Jo.

I know now that hurting people hurt people. Jo had been badly wounded over the many years she had been trying to make our family situation work; she felt that we had never really accepted her.

I thank God that I know this now. Back then, though, I didn't understand any of it.

The next morning we awoke early. I had the kids packed up and ready to go by six a.m. We drove down the driveway before Dad and Jo were awake and headed back to Cronulla.

8

I have walked and prayed for this young child an hour
And heard the sea-wind scream upon the tower …

— W.B. Yeats, 'A Prayer for my Daughter'

Giving birth to my child is one of the most amazing things I have ever done. I had dreamt of being a mother all my life: of nurturing a little person, being needed and loved unconditionally in a world that was stifled by conditions.

Maxwell Danger Rogers was born on 5 June 2006 by emergency Caesarian. The 'Danger' part was his father's idea; he figured it would help him pick up chicks when he was older.

I was induced two weeks early because I had a liver condition called obstetric cholestasis (or OC for short). An imbalance of bile salts made my skin feel as though it was crawling; I could not stop itching. It was very uncomfortable, but more importantly the doctor was concerned the baby might be affected — with OC, the risk of the baby being stillborn increases if the pregnancy goes to full term. Although it wasn't really a major consideration at the time, if we hadn't agreed to an emergency C-section Max could have arrived on 06/06/06, and we certainly didn't want to doom him from the start.

Max came into this world to the sound of Bon Jovi's 'Living on a Prayer', which was playing on the radio in the operating room. I'll never forget it; I was so out of it on the drugs they had given me I was singing along at the top of my voice:

'We're halfway there, oh, oh, living on a prayer!'

I was numb from the epidural, but I could feel my body being pulled around behind the sheet they had put up to shield me from the sight of my own abdomen being cut open. The doctor was talking Mat and I through what they were doing.

'OK, I can feel the head,' he said. Under the edge of the sheet screen I could just see him shifting his weight from one foot to the other.

'What is it, Doctor?' Mat asked expectantly. We were both really hoping for a boy. I know Mat especially wanted one. We had often shared our dreams of another boy to follow in his dad's and his granddad's sporting footsteps.

I could hear a small squeaky noise coming from the other side of the screen.

'It's a Wallaby,' the doctor said, lowering the sheet for us to see our newborn baby boy. Mat and I began to cry with joy as our baby was placed in my arms.

* * *

It amazed me, this tiny, perfect creature that was created inside my body. Every little finger and toe I was responsible for looking after — and believe me, I was extremely protective.

It's hard to convey even a part of the pain of finding out that your son, your first-born, the angel that you had nursed for those many months and watched grow, is never going to be the same as other kids. I used to daydream about him accomplishing great things in sport like his dad, going to school, getting married — all the usual things. My dreams were short-lived.

Max was such a perfect baby. He hardly ever made a noise and he slept so well. He was so easy; he would go to anyone and sleep through everything. My friends kept praising me, saying I had done such a good job with him. I felt truly blessed.

A few days after Max was born, Mat had to go back into Wallaby camp. He had flown down from the training camp at Coffs Harbour for Max's birth, and he had to go straight back into lockdown for pre-season training. Not long after that, Mat had to leave for Europe on the Wallabies tour. Luckily I had my amazing mum and grandma, who both moved in with me to help out.

I really struggled after Max's birth: for several weeks I was in a lot of pain from the emergency caesar. Breastfeeding was excruciating too at first, but I persevered because I wanted to do it so much. For the first three months, I barely left the house. What with feeds every few hours and pain from major abdominal surgery, I didn't even try.

One morning I was in bed feeding Max when I heard footsteps coming up the stairs. Suddenly the door burst open and there was my sister Camilla.

'What the –' I exclaimed as Camilla jumped into the bed with me and gave me a big hug. Tears fell down my face, I was so shocked but delighted to see her.

'Surprise!' Camilla said, and I saw mum standing in the doorway behind her. 'I flew her in from New York as a surprise,' Mum said with the biggest smile on her face.

'And this must be little Maxi,' Camilla said, stroking his tiny bald head. I finished feeding him and passed him gently across for a cuddle.

'This is Max and he is destined for greatness,' I said, staring adoringly at this little being that Mat and I had created.

'Max, this is Aunty Camilla,' I gestured to my sister. She fell instantly in love with him. Camilla had never been maternal — in fact, this would have to be the first time I'd ever seen her hold a baby — but right from the start there was a very special bond between Camilla and her little nephew.

After those first six weeks I was able to drive again, so I did get out a little. But our home was the hub of my existence at that time: Jack and Skyla would come and stay often and we would talk on Skype to Mat over in Europe before I dropped them at school. I wasn't working, thank God, so I could juggle a newborn with the older two kids. I always loved the idea of a big family, so I adored having them around. It was such a special time for them to be part of, too, getting to know their new little brother.

When Mat came back from playing overseas, he quickly slotted back into life with our new son. I think he hadn't found it easy to be so far away from home at this special time in our lives. Both of us had always known that constant travel and training were just part of the job, though — and thank God for Skype, which made it easier to stay in touch.

Then one day, I heard Mat answer the phone downstairs. It had to be one of his mates, I could tell from the tone of his voice, but I couldn't hear quite what he was saying. I came down the stairs with Max in my arms. I had just got him up for a feed and I was still in my pyjamas. I had taken to wearing tracksuits to bed, so that if I hadn't got round to getting dressed when people visited it didn't look as though I was still in my pyjamas, even though I was.

'Yeah, alright, what time?' Mat turned around from the windows overlooking the bay and I shrugged my shoulders inquiringly, trying to find out who it was.

'I will. Speak soon.' He hung up the phone.

'That was Mick,' he said. Mick was one of his mates from Cronulla. I had met him a few times and I got along really well with his wife Jaquie. We were both evil stepmums (as we called ourselves), so we had a lot in common.

'He wants me to go meet with this guy at the Sheraton to talk about maybe being part of this new rugby league team they are forming up on the Gold Coast.' I knew that look — he was excited.

This would be a big move for Mat — not just geographically, but it meant returning to league after switching across to union five years before.

'When is the meeting?' I asked, concerned that he might just jump into something without reading the fine print and weighing it up properly. He was known for doing that.

'Tomorrow,' Mat replied.

'Well, just make sure you don't sign anything straight away. If there's a contract, bring it back and I'll get Dad to look at it first.' He nodded, turning back to gaze across the bay. A ferry was slowly cruising by.

My whole family worked in law, so ever since I was a kid starting out in modelling I was taught not to sign anything right away, and there was always someone around to give me free legal advice. It was very handy, I must say.

'The Gold Coast, hey,' Mat murmured to himself, a slight smile playing across his face. Mat had grown up on the Gold Coast and I knew he had very fond memories of it. I just hoped they wouldn't cloud his thinking when it came to making a decision that would affect the whole family.

The next day he left early for his meeting in town. In between feeds, I spent the day wondering what was going on, until finally I got the phone call I was waiting for.

'Better pack your bags, darling, we're moving to the Gold Coast!' He almost sang down the phone.

'What? I told you not to sign anything!' I barked.

'Darling, the money is good — well, good enough, and I just think we need to get away from Cronulla.' He was firm with me in a loving way. I knew what he meant. Between Mat's divorce and Steve's death, Cronulla didn't hold that many happy memories for us. It is a very insular suburb so everyone knows everyone else's business, which makes it hard to escape from the past.

The money was irrelevant, really: it was less than Mat was being paid to play union but we would cash in on lifestyle up there — for us and especially for the kids. We would have to fly Jack and Skyla up from Sydney regularly; it would be difficult, but we knew they would absolutely love it up there.

Just as we were planning an escape from the black clouds of the recent past, new storms appeared on the horizon for our family.

It was 8 December 2006, eleven months after Steve's passing. With the loss of his father, Mat's brother Don had spiralled out of control. Often I would get calls from Danny, who would be hysterical because of the state Don was in. Their daughter Eden had been born just two months before and Don's erratic behaviour was creating a serious strain on their relationship. I was finding it very difficult to stay neutral: Don was Mat's brother, so he would always be part of our lives, but with Danny calling me all the time to fill me in on what he was up to, I began getting angry and less tolerant of Donny's dramas. I didn't want to feel like that, though: Don was my partner's brother and I just had to love him unconditionally.

I had just put Max down. He was six months old now and sleeping and eating so well. I absolutely loved being a mum — he made it easy for me to enjoy it all. I just assumed he was by nature a great baby: he wasn't freaked out by noise, he was really placid — I don't think he ever really cried. As a new mother my 'bible' was a book called *Baby Love* by Robin Barker. All my friends would say, 'I have to get that book because your baby is so good.' I look back now and wonder if these were all early signs that there was something different with Max.

It was the end of football season, so Mat was in Moree enjoying some well-earned R&R at a pub owned by our neighbour, Downsy. Early the next morning they were apparently going pig hunting, of all things. So Max and I were at home on our own. I quite liked the time Maxi and I had to ourselves, so it was no big deal. I knew Mat would have a ball with his mates and after working so hard all season, he deserved it.

Just as I went to sit down on the couch the phone began to ring. I smiled, figuring it would be Mat with a few beers under his belt. But it was Danny; her voice was shaking with fear.

'Hey, sweetie, what's wrong?' I walked out onto the verandah so my voice wouldn't wake Max.

'It's Don. He's threatening to kill himself.' Although she was clearly worried, there was exhaustion in her voice too from this psychological warfare that just never seemed to stop. This wasn't the first time Don had threatened to do something like this.

'I don't know what to do or who else to call,' she said desperately.

'Don't worry about him, we'll sort it out,' I tried to calm her, feeling angry that we were being put in such a situation but worried too that Don might do something stupid.

I hung up and dialled Mat's number. 'Hello darling,' Mat's husky voice rumbled in my ear, an edge of intoxication to it. In the background I could hear a lot of men laughing and carrying on.

'Darling, Danny just called. Apparently Don is going to commit suicide tonight.'

Mat shushed the men in the background. 'Shut up for a minute, will ya!' The background noise subsided.

'Should we ring the police or do you want to call him?' I asked, thinking it would be best if we just called the cops straight away.

I could picture Mat shaking his head at the absurdity of the whole thing. 'I'll ring him now then I'll call you back,' he said. And with that he hung up the phone.

Whatever the problem was with Don, I knew that Mat would be the one who could sort it out. I went back to my criminal investigation show on TV and ended up falling asleep on the couch. Several hours later I awoke, wondering what time it was. Mat had not called back, so everything must have been OK. I took myself upstairs to bed.

The next morning I got up and went about our daily routine. Max had had his breakfast and was playing in his little activity station, a circular device with a seat in the middle where he could turn around and play with different toys. I was sitting on the couch with a coffee, staring at my beautiful little man in a daze, when the phone rang. It was the police. They had been trying to call Mat, but he must have been out of range, hunting pigs somewhere near Moree. There had been an incident with his brother Don: apparently Danny had called off their relationship and left with baby Eden to go and stay at her mother's place. With the anniversary of his father's death looming, plus the first Christmas without his dad around, Don had reached a point where he felt the need to end it all. Danny had been worried for his wellbeing and had asked one of Don's friends to go and check on him. He found Don in real trouble, having taken a cocktail of prescription drugs and alcohol. His friend managed to drive Don to the hospital, where he was being treated for an overdose.

Mat was out of range still, so it was up to me to go and survey the damage. I got off the phone with the police and immediately called Mum. I always called her in a crisis. She would know what to do.

'Mum, it's Donny — he's tried to kill himself.' A sense of helplessness mixed with a whole lot of other emotions suddenly hit me and the tears started. I felt quite overwhelmed, dealing with this without Mat by my side.

'What? Oh, my God!' she said, clearly shocked. 'Where is he?'

'He's in hospital, I have to go see him. Mat's not back from Moree till tonight. I was wondering if you could look after Maxi for me?'

'Oh, darling, I'm on a train on my way to work,' Mum replied.

'It's OK, I'll just take him with me.'

'What a mess! It's just been one thing after another,' she exclaimed.

'I know.' I was beginning to think life with a Rogers was never going to be without drama.

'OK, well, keep me posted,' she said.

Hanging up the phone I took a deep breath and prepared myself for the day ahead. I was going to have to go to the Sutherland Hospital psychiatric ward with a six-month-old in tow.

When I arrived at the hospital there were some police around the entrance to the ward, but thankfully no paparazzi. I pushed Max in his pram to the big front entrance and then through the glass doors. As I walked in, the lady at the reception desk eyed Max and I curiously in between clicking keys on a computer.

'Hello, we're here to see Don Rogers — he was admitted earlier on today,' I said confidently, hoping she wouldn't twig to who I was. I was reluctant to help sell any more papers with a Rogers family drama. Already this year, we had lost Steve, begun the process of a divorce settlement with Mat's ex-wife, decided to move interstate, changed football codes, had an emergency

C-section — and now this, an attempted suicide. It had honestly been an *annus horribilis*, as Queen Elizabeth II would say.

The receptionist buzzed us through a heavy-duty door and led us into the ward. I walked through, cautiously looking from left to right. There appeared to be some pretty intense people around. One lady was having a conversation with herself in the corner of the room, her face pressed up against the wall, as though she were communicating through it to someone on the other side. A gentleman appeared to be hysterically singing to another, who on closer inspection was snoring, fast asleep.

'Welcome to the Sutherland psych ward, honey, plenty of entertainment for you in here,' the receptionist said, sensing my unabashed curiosity.

'This is Donald's room.' She gestured to one of the many doors that lined the hall.

'Thank you,' I said and quietly crept in. Don was lying on his bed reading a book.

'Hey, mate, how's it going?' I asked, trying to sound cheerful as I looked around at the pokey little room with its bare walls.

'Hey, Chloe, I'm good now, thanks. How are you?' Don slowly got off the bed and came to greet us with a cuddle. He looked pale and nervy: I was pretty sure a little of whatever he had taken was still in his system.

'Do you mind if we go outside for a cigarette?' This was not going to be easy for Don to talk about; I guess he figured a stimulant of some sort might help him get through it.

'Sure,' I said, liking the idea of being outside even though I didn't smoke any more.

We walked out to the smoking area and found a bench to sit on. Max was fast asleep in his pram. Observing some of the other patients out there, I was a little uneasy. Although we were outside, the brick walls were very high.

Don fumbled a cigarette from the pack then asked a girl nearby if she had a light. She offered him one then walked off toward the wall behind us. I watched as she took something out of her pocket that looked like a calculator. She pressed a few keys then lifted it to her ear, and began to converse as though it were a mobile phone. I was intrigued to see how long she would keep it up.

Meanwhile Donny had lit his cigarette and was staring straight ahead, deep in thought.

'What happened, mate?' I asked, keeping my eye on the calculator girl as Don took a deep breath and relayed his perspective of events.

I listened and nodded as I rocked little Maxi's pram. I was ready if anyone came near him to attack. I think everyone was on medication, though, as they all seemed pretty docile.

I listened to Don for over half an hour, interjecting where I thought appropriate and trying to be positive. The last thing I wanted was to make him feel guilty for being here. Donny told me of his struggle with his mother's death, his father's death, and now potentially the loss of his daughter and partner. Understandably he was an emotional wreck, but I felt sure that he was doing OK and in the best place possible. My concern now was how Mat was going to take it all.

Finally it was time to leave and I hugged Donny and said goodbye. Wheeling my pram back through that heavy door, I asked to see his doctor before I left, so I could make sure Mat could contact him when he finally heard the news. This was all arranged; the doctor gave me his direct line.

Outside the ward I tried phoning Mat again. Finally he picked up.

'Hi, darling,' he sounded cheerful but a bit dusty.

'Darling, I've got some bad news. Don tried to commit suicide and he's now in the psych ward at Sutherland Hospital,' I said, half expecting him to lose it on the phone.

'Oh my God — you're kidding!' he exclaimed.

'I'm just leaving the psych ward now. He seems OK but I think they want to keep him in here for a little while.' I had told the doctor I thought this would be a really good idea. I passed on the doctor's details to Mat so he could get an update on Don's progress.

'I need you to get on a plane back straight away,' I said.

'OK, I'll sort something out,' he said and hung up the phone.

Mat got back and went to see Don that night. He managed to slip past the paparazzi that were lurking outside by now. Someone working at the hospital had alerted the papers.

The doctors wanted to keep Don in for up to a week. I wasn't sure if it would be enough.

Quite frankly, I couldn't wait for 2006 to be over.

9

'A woman can be proud and stiff
When on love intent;
But Love has pitched his mansion in
The place of excrement;
For nothing can be sole or whole
That has not been rent.'

— W.B. Yeats, 'Crazy Jane Talks with the Bishop'

Like most families, Christmas is a very special time for us but it comes with its own little giftwrapped bundle of challenges. This time of year, everyone wants a piece of the kids, and it can be quite a juggling act when you've got several branches of family spread around the country.

We were gearing up to make the big move up to the Gold Coast. We had decided to move at the end of January, so Mat and I had been trawling the internet looking for a new home. We had a long list of places that we were planning to check out after the Christmas and New Year celebrations.

At this time of year we would often go to Palm Beach, Sydney's northernmost suburb on a peninsula jutting into the ocean, to visit my dad's side of the family.

Ever since we were kids and my mum and dad separated, we would spend every second Christmas there. This year, my dad and Jo had hired a house at Palm Beach for a week over the Christmas period. At the last minute, we decided we would spend some time with them before our move. My Uncle Tony has a beautiful big place in Byron Bay, so we were planning to head up after Boxing Day and celebrate New Year's Eve there. From there, we could drive an hour or so up to the Gold Coast and look for somewhere to live.

It was a well-laid plan, but I must say it turned out to be one of our more difficult Christmases.

Max was six months old now, and I had just weaned him. I was excited that I could have a few drinks with my family and not have to worry about the effects they would have on my breast milk and consequently on Maxi. In my family, having a glass of wine with dinner is part of the fabric of life, especially on social occasions, and it would be nice to be part of that again.

I wasn't at all worried about Max being unsettled in a strange place: he was always so happy and easygoing, never fazed by much. Everyone just thought he was the perfect child: he would go to anyone and he never had trouble sleeping. We could have a dinner party downstairs with the music on and he wouldn't wake.

The house that Dad and Jo rented in Palm Beach was beautiful but not terribly practical for a six-month-old child to be crawling around in but it was a last-minute decision on our part to come, so it wasn't originally rented to accommodate us. It had polished wooden floorboards and a great big staircase leading from the entrance level to the one below where the bedrooms were.

My stepsister Erin would be staying at the Palm Beach house too, together with her boyfriend at the time. Erin was a gorgeous girl with blue eyes and long blonde hair. Sadly, we had never been especially close growing up. I was fourteen when she came onto the scene as a nine-year-old. Brodie, Camilla and I were desperately jealous of her as kids because she had her own bedroom and we were forced to sleep on bunk beds. Looking back now, it was so silly: she spent a lot more time at Dad and Jo's house, so of course she would have her own room. But kids are funny; great recorders not great interpreters.

Back then, Erin was known for running away from home frequently. She had suffered terribly with the breakup of her parents so she was a very rebellious presence in the household as we were growing up. Despite all of these issues she has grown into a beautiful woman; I am so proud of how far she has come and constantly amazed at how well she can deal with things now.

Also staying with us in Palm Beach were my brother Brodie and his then-fiancée Kate. They had met many moons ago working for Tyrrell's Wines; Brodie is a graphic designer and Kate is in marketing and sales. They are just the cutest couple and the rest of the family absolutely adore Kate. She had really made a massive difference to my little brother. Brodie was never very motivated and he was quite happy just coasting along in life until he met Kate. She inspired him to do better, to strive for more — which is what a partner should do, I believe. Corny though it might sound, I often think he was just waiting for Kate to come along to complete him.

Christmas Eve was a lovely day; as the breeze played in the palm trees, we all piled into two cars and wound our way up the meandering streets of Palm Beach to my grandparents' house. We all called my grandparents 'Bups' and 'Gugs': as a child my cousin Amy couldn't pronounce 'Grandma' and 'Grandpa' properly so the names just stuck.

All of us were there that morning except Mat. His training for the Gold Coast Titans would only finish that afternoon, giving him a six-week break over the holiday period. He also had some last-minute packing to do for our big move. He would drive down first thing in the morning to join us and he would really want to unwind. It was Michelle's turn to have Jack and Skyla this Christmas, so it would just be Mat, Max and myself.

We rounded the last bend on the road and arrived at my grandparents' house. They had lived in this house for as long as I had been alive, a beautiful two-storey place with immaculate gardens. My grandmother had always been into her gardening. It was a passion that all her children shared — both the gardening and the quest for perfection, which manifested in many different areas of their lives, sometimes to their detriment. Everything can't be perfect all of the time, so for anyone who wants it that way, life can be stressful.

As we walked up the steep slope, I had a flashback to the time my dad left his car in the driveway and forgot to put the handbrake on. Some very disgruntled neighbours came knocking that day to ask him to remove his car from their lounge room. My dad is an incredibly smart man, a talented barrister — and yet he is a klutz, so things like this often happen to him. I think that's where I got it from. His wife, Jo, is slightly klutzy too, so they seemed to suit each other.

Jo and I had never really seen eye to eye since that fateful night in Rydal. We had talked and worked a few things out but there was still plenty of uneasiness between us. I was a fourteen-year-old girl when she was introduced to me as my dad's new girlfriend all those years ago. I was extremely overprotective of my mother so it must have been really hard for Jo from the beginning. Back then, I don't think she really felt comfortable with any of us kids. We often thought she couldn't wait to be rid of us so she could just spend time with Dad. Looking back, we were absolute little monsters, so I'm not surprised that she may have felt that way.

We walked up the steps to the house, weighed down with food, alcohol, baby essentials and presents. I was carrying Max: everyone was more excited to see him than me, which is very often the case with babies.

We spent the day enjoying great food and fine wine — two things that always go hand in hand at any Maxwell occasion. This stretched well into the evening. My cousin Amy had offered to look after Max; she wasn't interested in having a big night as she had a little one too, Cooper, and so I was free to drink and be merry. I was very excited but a bit nervous as well. I hadn't had much freedom since having Max. I would either end up coming home early because I was too tired, or I would totally obliterate myself on alcohol.

It ended up being the latter. Unfortunately I must have thought I could still stomach the same amount of alcohol I drank before I had a child.

Mat arrived early on Christmas morning to find a very dishevelled, very hung-over me. I had managed to pull myself up out of bed and empty the contents of my stomach several times before he had arrived. The bedroom was dark and smelt of alcohol as he crept in.

'Good morning, darling, merry Christmas,' he said, seating himself on the side of the bed.

'Eurgh,' was about all I could manage.

'Whoa! You look terrible. Big night?'

Wiping the saliva from the side of my face and parting my matted hair just enough to peer through it with one eye, I gave him an evil stare.

'Looks like it. Ha ha!'

He was very amused to see me in such a state. It had been a year and a half since I had had a big night, whereas he had many such nights without the worry of being pregnant or breastfeeding. I was fast realising this drinking stuff was very overrated.

Mat's phone began to ring. The sound made me feel nauseous, but I peered at the phone through my hair to see who was calling. It was Michelle.

'Hello?' Mat answered, then listened intently for a minute. He always braced himself for one drama or another when she called.

'OK.' He hung up and got to his feet. 'I have to go get the kids from the Central Coast. Michelle wants us to have them now.'

I opened my mouth to say something but the sound of the door upstairs opening and closing distracted me. Max's baby noises could be heard, along with the sound of Dad and Jo fussing over him. They must have gone to pick him up from Amy for me.

'Slowly scraping myself up out of bed. I shuffled up the stairs, trying not to shake my brain in my head too much with each step.

'Well, hello, sunshine!' Dad had a great sense of humour, which was even greater when it was not directed at me.

'Hi,' I said croakily, walking as though I had just had major brain surgery.

'So the kids are coming over?' Jo asked, picking a banana out of the fruit bowl, peeling it and handing it to Max.

'Yeah, Michelle just rang.' I sat down at the kitchen table, massaging my temples. Max took the banana and began eating it carefully, making sure only to touch the skin and not the flesh with his fingers. I had always thought that slightly odd.

'Yeah — sorry, this is what we have to deal with, I'm afraid,' I replied. Nothing more was said and the kids were fine once they got there. We were fast running out of space at the rental, though, so I asked my grandparents if we could spend one night in the self-contained unit at their place before we left.

That night we put the kids down and watched a little tennis on TV with my grandparents. We were engrossed in the match when my phone rang. It was my brother Brodie.

'Hi, Chloe, it's me.' Brodie's voice sounded unusual; I could sense the hostility.

'What's wrong?' I asked.

'I am that pissed off right now!' He spat down the phone. 'Is there room for us to stay there tonight? Can you ask Gugs and Bups?'

I looked over at Bups nodding off on the couch. Next to him Gugs was still avidly watching the tennis.

'Gugs?' I asked in between rallies.

'Yes, dear?' she replied.

'Is there room for Brodie and Kate to come and stay tonight?' I asked, knowing the answer already.

'Of course there is, darling, they can have the upstairs section of the flat.' I vaguely remembered Brodie and Dad having an argument on the boat he had gone out on that day. Perhaps that had escalated, I thought to myself.

When Brodie and Kate arrived, I asked them what was going on.

'Jo wanted to give us advice on marriage!' Brodie spat, clearly upset.

I looked at Kate, who nodded silently. She was never one for confrontation.

I ushered them inside and listened to their angry rants most of the night.

The following day I was ready to go into battle for them. We drove down with the kids in the car to pick up some bits and pieces we had left in the house. Seeing Jo as we arrived, I launched into her.

'How dare you think you can give Kate and Brodie advice on marriage!' I was so angry. Their issues combined with my issues with Jo were fuelling me now and there was no stopping me.

'How can you give them advice on marriage when you're on your second?' I was just getting warmed up.

'I was trying to protect Kate,' she said, quivering with anger.

I began to cry suddenly, feeling exhausted from all of the fighting and bickering.

'Why does this have to happen? We've had such a lovely time together. I hate fighting!'

Dad appeared from down the stairs.

'What's going on, Dad?' I asked.

'I agree with Jo,' he said matter-of-factly.

With that I turned on my heel, jumped in the car and we left.

Immediately following my brother's wedding in March, I felt it necessary to send Dad a 12-page email voicing my disapproval of his conduct from the time of my parents' separation.

I didn't speak to my dad again for over a year. All of our years of pent-up emotion had finally come to a head in what would be the biggest metamorphosis in our relationship. It was not easy but looking back now, I can see that it was necessary.

10

For everything that's lovely is
But a brief, dreamy, kind delight.

— W.B. Yeats, 'Never Give All the Heart'

I can't say how grateful we were to be able to close the door on 2006 and start 2007 afresh in a different state, with Mat playing a different code of football. Everything seemed new and the future was full of hope.

The press were having a field day with Mat's switch back to rugby league. It was a seriously big deal. People were particularly fired up by the fact that he had terminated his contract with the Wallabies just before they competed in the World Cup. Perhaps they would have done better if he had been there — it was not their finest cup performance, being knocked out in the semifinal.

Signing Mat was considered a major coup for the new league team they called the Jetstar Gold Coast Titans. The Coast was abuzz with the birth of this new team. There is something about Queenslanders that sets them apart: there's a sense of pride and a real camaraderie that shows through in times like the floods that swept through the state in early 2011. The way the state banded together in one of the most devastating times of our history was simply awe-inspiring. Complete strangers helped each other rebuild their lives. If only all families acted the same.

We were living on a canal initially, in Florida Gardens. A canal system loops through the Gold Coast, weaving its way from north to south. I thought it strange at first that people actually lived on these man-made canals, with so many other houses directly opposite. Some of the canals weren't very wide: you could literally throw a stone from one side to the other. But the quality of life in Queensland was so much better. I couldn't believe that we were paying less rent than we had in Cronulla yet we were right on the water. We absolutely loved it, and so did the kids. Every morning Jack would be out front at sunrise, checking the crab pot or dropping a line in. He would often have made a decent catch before the rest of the household woke.

We really hoped that we might buy that house one day, but those dreams were squashed when we received notice that the owner had decided to sell the place. We were understandably upset, as we had discussed with the agent the possibility of eventually buying it direct from the owner. Next thing we knew, people began to filter through for a stickybeak. To the average person that's quite a normal experience, but when your face has been plastered all over the local paper for the past few months, it's a little different. There was absolutely no privacy: the estate agent was telling potential buyers who lived there, and I swear some of Mat's undies went missing.

So we got out of there pretty quickly and ended up buying a place in Clear Island Waters, a beautiful area set beside a freshwater lake. Our house wasn't in the best location but it was nicely renovated and all on one level, which was perfect for our growing little family. It also had a big backyard, though as we later discovered, it was infested with green ants. These things give the most painful bites that swell up into welts. I don't know what was worse — the sandflies while we were living on the water or the green ants on the dry block. Small prices to pay for such great places to live, I suppose.

The biggest surprise was that I was expecting again. We had wanted to have another baby — Mat was all for me just churning them out — but I didn't think it would happen so soon after the first. I had only just finished breastfeeding Max when I fell pregnant again.

Max was developing pretty much like any other little boy. His first word was 'car' and we thought that was such a typical boy thing. Indeed, he was quite obsessed with cars. He would line them up and push them around for hours, watching their wheels turn ever so closely. My brother is still obsessed over cars even as an adult, so I didn't think it was that abnormal.

I remember a time when Maxi used to engage with me, when he would look me in the eye. We used to say, 'Show us your muscles,' and he would proudly display his little muscles just like Daddy taught him.

After he turned one, though, it was as though he started to go backwards. Max no longer looked anyone in the eye; he never showed his muscles when we asked — in fact, our requests would be met with a blank stare. He didn't even acknowledge that it was something he was familiar with.

There was a time when Max used to laugh uncontrollably at things that tickled his sense of the ridiculous. If he was watching a cartoon and someone fell over, he thought it was hysterical. One time we were travelling to a function; Jack and Skyla were with us and Max was in his baby seat. Skyla threw her phone up and it hit the roof, and Max just started laughing so hard, we didn't think he would stop. So then it was all on. We just kept throwing various things up to make him laugh, because it was so delightful to see him just bursting with giggles. When Max was around eighteen months, it stopped. Quite suddenly he no longer laughed at all of the things that used to amuse him so much.

Max became more and more fascinated with the most mundane things. Quite early one morning I heard a noise in the kitchen. Mat had already gone to training — I was used to that. The Clear Island Waters house was an L shape, with our bedroom at one end of the house and Max's at the other. I tiptoed out in my nightie, half expecting a burglar, and found Max stacking baked bean cans on the kitchen floor with a glazed look in his eye. It was spooky. I remember thinking he looked as though the lights were on but no one was home. One by one he put one can on top of another inside the pantry door. I watched him for some time without him even turning to look at me. Was my son possessed? What was this?

Max was my first baby, and I was at home alone with him every day while my husband was training long hours. After playing rugby union for five years, Mat was finding that first year back in the NRL very tough. I had no family on the coast and nothing else to compare Max to. Jack and Skyla were well past that toddler stage when I first met them. We had had so much drama in our lives over the past eighteen months that I guess we weren't noticing — or more to the point, I wasn't noticing — Max's lack of communication and interaction with other people. I really just thought that his behaviour was normal for him, that it was just Max.

Our house on Clear Island Waters had a pool and Max used to love being around it so he could throw things in the water and watch them as they sank. The pool had regulation fencing, though, so Max could only get in there with adult supervision. One day I came out to find Max lying on his stomach, studying the bottom of one of the poles in the fence. Looking closer, I noticed his little fingers were unscrewing one of the bolts. I bent down to scold him and noticed another three bolts lying beside him on the ground. I was dumbfounded. He had obviously wanted to get into the pool area so badly that he had methodically undone one of the poles bolt by bolt to get under the fence. I thought he was a genius and would surely be a remarkable mechanic.

The signs were there that Maxi was an unusual little boy. I just did not want to see or believe them — and I sure as hell didn't want any smug doctors telling me there was something wrong with my precious boy.

Mat's rugby league career with the Titans kicked off in their first game ever on the Gold Coast, a trial match against the Penrith Panthers.

I had scored myself a gig on Sea FM, the Gold Coast's local radio station, presenting my own show on Saturday mornings, called *Footballers' Wives*. I found it hilarious that my media repertoire had now expanded to include football, given my significant lack of expertise in the field. But I was married to a footballer, so that apparently gave me inside knowledge.

I had also been given a role on the live outside broadcast the station would do from every Titans home game. Leading up to the game we would do a two-hour show including interviews with players and coaches — like a warm-up but on radio.

The team's inaugural home ground was an old AFL (Australian Rules) stadium in Carrara. It was quite worn down and not an easy place to watch play, having been designed for a totally different style of football. Our outside broadcast was set up in the car park, a dusty paddock at the side of the stadium. My co-host and the show's producer, Jason, and I would be interviewing some injured players and some fans as they entered the gates.

'Do you think we could get an interview with Mat?' my producer asked a couple of days before the match.

'I'll try,' I replied, not wanting to upset my boss before the first show. I knew that Mat didn't like doing interviews before a game, especially if he was playing. It was as if he was a different person on game day. He would very rarely speak to me. He could be mistaken for being angry, but inside his head he was preparing to do battle. He had to be focused and ready: when he ran out on to the field that afternoon, it wasn't just to kick a ball around for some laughs. He would be faced by big men. Men who were often twice his size. Men who wanted to hurt him as much as their incredible strength and the rules of the game would allow.

Which was why I was so surprised when he agreed to an interview.

'Sure I'll do one. What time do you want me there?' He asked in a strangely upbeat tone for someone about to play their first real game back in rugby league.

'Is four o'clock OK?' I asked, and he nodded in reply. Our show started at four and went all the way up to kick-off at six, so Mat's interview would be at the head of the show.

A handful of die-hard fans were milling around the car park as we prepared for the show. It was still two and half hours to kick-off and too early for most of the spectators to be there yet.

We were standing on a big black stage with Sea FM signage

all around it. There were three of us: Galey, one of the station's favourite jocks, Jason the producer and program director of the station, and me. All three of us were decked out in black shirts with Sea FM and Titans logos embroidered on them, our standard wear for outside broadcasts. Mat had actually ironed my shirt for me, which was an unusual thing for him to do that morning.

Four o'clock began to loom closer and I had my eye out for Mat. He was supposed to be here for the beginning of the show; this was my first-ever gig for these guys, so I was very nervous. I was beginning to have flashbacks to the day we met. Was he going to show support for me this time or would I be left standing there like a tool once again? Sitting on the black stage under the black canopy, sweat began to form across my forehead.

'Man, it's hot.' I turned to Jason. He was distracted, on the phone teeing up our phone interviews for the show. None of my workmates knew I was pregnant. For starters I was not yet twelve weeks pregnant, so it wasn't public knowledge yet; I was also worried they wouldn't give me the job if they knew. I had specifically gone after a radio job because I knew once I had proven my worth it wouldn't matter if I became pregnant or not. I could be the size of a house and do radio.

I raised my eyes to see Mat's familiar frame sauntering towards us. 'Thank God,' I whispered under my breath.

'Mat's here.' I nudged Jason, who instantly hung up the phone with an excited schoolboy look in his eyes. Galey leapt up to shake Mat's hand and welcome him to the stage. Over the years I'd seen this reaction many times from boys and men alike. I often forgot that Mat was a hero to so many.

He shook their hands and gave me a big smooch on the lips. A crowd of fans magically materialised at the front of the stage, their eyes fixed on Mat, waiting to hang off every word he said.

'OK, we're going live in two minutes,' Jason said, prompting us all to put on headphones so that we could hear the live feed. I handed Mat a pair.

'Are you nervous?' he asked me.

'Yes,' I said, trying to focus on the questions I was going to ask him.

'So am I,' he whispered. I figured he was talking about the game.

The pre-recorded opener played and then we were on. 'Hello and welcome to Sea FM's pre-game show coming to you live from Carrara, where the mighty Jetstar Gold Coast Titans take on the Penrith Panthers in their first-ever home game. I'm Jason, and hello to Galey and Chloe Maxwell.' We said a quick hello then threw to a song. Next up would be our interview with Mat.

The song ended and Jason began. 'Joining us now is one of the most talked about signings of the Jetstar Titans and Chloe's other half — Mat Rogers, welcome.' The fans went absolutely mental with applause. The crowd had quadrupled since we had first arrived.

'Thanks for having me,' Mat said in his typically humble way.

'Now, Mat, it's a big game for you — returning after your stint in rugby union, playing the Panthers today. Can you walk us through how you prepare yourself for a game like this?' Galey was on fire with the sporty questions. I was yet to say anything, paralysed with nerves. Mat was sheer confidence.

'Well, my preparations on game day would include Chloe. She is very good to me and ...' He got down on one knee and pulled a little box out of his Titans shorts pocket. As he opened it I could see an amazing diamond ring sparkling in the sunlight. 'Today I would like to ask her if she would marry me.'

I swallowed hard, absolutely shocked with what I was witnessing — with what thousands of people on the radio and at the stadium were now witnessing.

'Oh my gosh, yes! Yes! Of course I'll marry you!' I was overcome with emotion as Mat slipped the ring onto my finger and got to his feet. I threw my arms around him.

'Wow, that was the sweetest thing I have ever witnessed on radio. We'll be right back after these messages.' Jason very professionally threw to commercials.

'I have to go and get ready now, darling,' Mat said, kissing me once more on the lips. 'I love you.' And with that he was gone, jogging away into the distance.

I struggled to get my act together after that, but I think my boss was pretty understanding. In fact I think he was over the moon that the first show had such newsworthy, water-cooler-deserving material.

11

Once more the storm is howling, and half hid
Under this cradle-hood and coverlid
My child sleeps on.

— W.B. Yeats, 'A Prayer for My Daughter'

On 19 September 2007, Phoenix Rogers, our beautiful daughter, was born. I was so ecstatic to have a baby girl and a baby boy — a pigeon pair. I felt blessed.

My mother had flown up from Sydney to be by my side, as she had done when Max was born. I was so aware of her support for both my births, and grateful for it. Between her and my eighty-year-old grandmother, meals were cooked, washing was done and our baby had all new clothes and the best of everything.

I was still not talking to Dad or to Jo, so they weren't invited to come and see their new granddaughter Phoenix. They couldn't have come anyway, as they were in Montpellier, having booked to see Mat play in the World Cup prior to his transfer to rugby league. She would be four months old before they would lay eyes on her.

My obstetrician had advised me to have an elective Caesarian as he felt that, at fifteen months apart, the two births were too close together to risk a natural delivery. To tell you the truth, I was quite happy with that. That way, I knew exactly what to expect. He told me I would come in to hospital at seven thirty and the baby would be out by nine. No hiccups.

Mat was with me as they were wheeling me into the operating room. He was so incredibly excited about having another baby and he was so supportive through it all. I, on the other hand, was quite frightened. I've never really felt comfortable around hospitals — any experiences I have had of them have been traumatic ones. Mat was the polar opposite: hospitals were something he had grown very comfortable with. Being a professional footballer, he was in and out of hospitals as regularly as most of us were in and out of the shower. Once when we were driving around Sydney, he pointed to each hospital we passed and said, 'That's where I had my knee reconstruction,' or 'That's where I had my shoulder fixed.' Kind of morbid, really.

Lying on the hospital bed waiting to be wheeled into the operating room, I mucked around with Mat, telling jokes and taking silly photos. I pretended to be a homie throwing a gang symbol: in the gown and shower cap with my big belly, it was hilarious.

I was beginning to get really nervous about the impending operation. The anaesthetist had already pricked me in several places with something to ensure I felt nothing. It was a scary sensation to be numb from the waist down and yet completely wide awake; I felt incredibly vulnerable.

One of the attending nurses entered the little room as Mat and I were whispering and giggling nervously. Looking down, I noticed she was carrying a large plastic bag and I was worried there would be more scary hospital stuff in there. I was wrong. She reached in and began to pull out handfuls of Jetstar Gold Coast Titans paraphernalia. For a moment I was sure I was hallucinating. I rubbed my eye with one hand while squeezing Mat's hand with the other. Glancing at him, I could see that he too seemed perplexed. Our gaping mouths didn't slow her down in the slightest, though, as she began taking out a seemingly endless stream of items one by one and placing them on my pregnant belly for Mat to sign.

I couldn't believe it — this woman had a complete disregard for our special moment. She carried on pulling out beanies, mugs, jerseys and footy cards with no shame whatsoever. I was mortified. I mean, who would do that? One autograph would have been OK, but she had obviously known we were coming in for months and had collected items from every living relative. Disgraceful!

Mat is such a lovely person. Instead of getting angry, he went right ahead and signed every last thing she shoved up his nose. If I could have felt my legs I would have kicked her right in the Titans mug!

The birth went very smoothly once we got past the initial nonsense. This time round, knowing exactly what I was in for helped to quell my fears. That was until I was wheeled into the operating theatre. Tears began to fill my eyes as I looked up at Mat. He was holding my hand and smiling ever so softly. He knew I was afraid. Childbirth is frightening at the best of times, let alone when you are lying on a table, still conscious, about to be cut open.

The mask was placed over my mouth as the anaesthetist worked to maintain my numbness. I felt my body being tugged behind the sheet the doctors and nurses hide behind so you are not freaked out by the sight of them cutting you open. I remember mumbling to Mat, 'I am never going through this again!' Then a rather large tug was accompanied by a very audible squeak.

'It's a girl!' The doctor and nurses chimed together as they dropped the sheet for me to see her.

Mat and I cried tears of joy. 'Our little girl,' I whispered softly to him as he kissed my forehead.

After the nurses had cleaned and weighed her, they brought our baby over swaddled in terry towelling for me to hold.

'Our little girl,' I whispered again, the tears spilling down my cheeks and onto the pillow.

It was school holidays and Jack and Skyla had been staying with us. The kids had had an absolute ball: they had been to all of the theme parks and we had done the movies, bowling and putt putt golf. Mat always tended to go overboard with the activities while the older kids were here because he missed them so much. It was what my dad used to do when we were kids and we went to his place every second weekend.

The last day before Jack and Skyla had to go back to Sydney, we went to Dreamworld. It was undoubtedly our favourite out of all of the 'Worlds'. Jack and I went on every scary ride a few times just to make sure they really were terrifying. Mat would always feign injury to avoid going on those rides. It's hilarious that he is completely comfortable running at men twice his size but goes weak at the knees at the thought of the 'Giant Drop'.

We had come home after a massive day. Before we could relax we needed to pack everything up, ready for Jack and Skyla to catch the plane home in the morning. I liked to make sure all the kids' clothes were clean and neatly folded to take home.

'Alright, guys, time to gather up all of your stuff so we can pack your bags,' I said, carrying Maxi through to the bath.

I had just turned off the tap when I heard a heated conversation coming from the kids' room.

'I don't want to go!' Jack was saying to his dad.

'What's going on?' I asked, poking my head around the door. I saw Jack curled up under his doona on the bed, clearly upset. Mat was sitting on the side of the bed.

'Jack doesn't want to go home tomorrow,' Mat replied, looking up at me with pain in his eyes.

'If you make me I'll run away,' Jack said, his tears staining the pillow.

I looked at Mat stroking Jack's hair and pondering what to

do. Skyla was sitting on her bed, shaking her head. She didn't seem to have any problems going home and was quite taken aback by Jack's behaviour.

'Well I don't want to make him if he doesn't want to go,' I said to Mat, suddenly feeling fiercely protective of him. I hated to see the kids hurt and upset.

Jack had the most incredible relationship with his dad, like most boys do with their dads. They really were like two peas in a pod. There was a special affinity between father and son that was irreplaceable. I believe it is so important that a father's connection with his son remains good and pure. Unconditional love is difficult when they misbehave, but it is so important for the child's future development. When that relationship becomes strained or lost it can lead to the demise of the child, emotionally and sometimes physically. That's why when a man sees a psychiatrist with their issues, the psychiatrist always wants to know what their relationship with their father was like.

'I don't want to put him on the plane,' I said finally, deciding to put my foot down. 'It's not a big deal if a boy wants to come and live with his dad. In fact that's quite normal I would imagine. Michelle would understand,' I said, turning and heading to the kitchen to make a cup of tea and work out exactly how this was going to happen.

'You might have to give your mum a call, mate, and explain it to her.' Mat's gentle voice travelled down the hall to the kitchen as I retrieved two mugs from the cupboard.

'No!' Jack was adamant. I could tell he was desperate not to hurt his mum's feelings.

'You can't just not show up at the airport, Jack — we have to let her know, otherwise you will have to get on that plane tomorrow,' Mat replied matter-of-factly.

'Why don't you both sleep on it and see how you go in the morning?' I suggested, pouring milk into both mugs of tea and feeling the steam caress my forehead as I leaned in to take a sip from one.

The next day both kids' bags were packed ready to go on the plane. It seemed as though Jack had decided to go home to his mum's house.

'Bye, sweetie, I love you.' I kissed Jack and gave him a hug.

'Bye, Skyla, honey.' We squeezed each other in a tight embrace.

An hour later Mat rang.

'He didn't get on the plane.' I could hear mixed emotions in his voice: happiness to have his son but anxiety about how Michelle was going to react. I anticipated she wasn't going to be very happy. I was right.

Looking back, it wasn't the best way to go about things. After having to go through the courts for Jack, we certainly learnt our lesson. The only people who really win in those situations are the lawyers.

Jack moved back to his mum's house after only six months with us. The pressure of living with his decision was a little too much for him to cope with, and his mother had been devastated by his choice.

In these months of custody battles over Jack, I hardly registered the fact my little boy Max was becoming more and more withdrawn. Our family struggles, along with Mat's career shift and the move to the Gold Coast, overshadowed everything else. One by one, none of those things are extraordinary, but all together it was perhaps enough to mask what was going on with Max.

More than that, though, I never imagined there might be something wrong with him. He'd had all his shots, been through all the usual tests, seen the paediatrician on schedule and everything was fine. He was in the ninety-eighth percentile for growth so as far as I was concerned, he was flourishing. You worry about your child being born with a congenital condition that will affect them for life, but I never really considered that he might develop anything a couple of years after being born. I simply didn't know that something like this could happen.

12

He, too, has resigned his part
In the casual comedy;
He, too, has been changed in his turn,
Transformed utterly …

— W.B. Yeats, 'Easter 1916'

What was it about live TV that kept drawing me back? I must be a glutton for punishment — it's not the easiest television to do, that's for sure. I loved it though. Flying by the seat of your pants, the thrill of never quite knowing what was going to happen next. It's a thrill that you don't get too often when you have two kids under the age of two. I guess there's the thrill of wondering whether or not their nappy will withstand a full-on bottom explosion, or if they might manage to keep down what they have eaten and not spray it all over you.

Several months after Phoenix was born, I was asked to audition for a show called *It Takes Two*. It was a reality show that had had reasonable success overseas and its first two seasons here in Australia were very well received. Celebrities were paired up with professional singers and they would then compete against each other, performing to a live audience every week. The real entertainment lay in the fact that most of the celebrities could not sing to save themselves. The people at home would vote for their favourites; a celebrity and their singing partner would be voted off every week until the final show, when the winners were revealed.

I flew down to my audition at Fox Studios in Sydney with the kids, who would spend the day with my mum. Even though it was hard work looking after two little ones Mum loved having them, so she jumped at the chance to take care of them for the day and to help me get back into some television work.

I had never balked at the idea of flying with the kids on my own. As long as I was prepared with treats, activities and a bottle (milk for the kids, not wine for me these days!) for take-off and landing, I knew I would be OK. Max was always very friendly with everyone on the plane, especially the flight attendants. He was so flirtatious; on one flight, I distinctly remember him searching over my shoulder for the hostess, locking his eyes on her with a big grin and waiting for her to come back.

This time was different. Loaded down with bags and the two little ones, I edged through to our seats. I took the aisle seat and put Phoenix on my lap, with Max in the window seat. He usually loved being by the window, but when we were settled in our seats he suddenly started to look around anxiously. His breathing began to sound very irregular.

'Are you OK, Maxi?' I asked as I put Phoenix onto my breast to feed. Max began kicking his feet against the seat in front and making loud grunting noises.

'Stop that, mate,' I said, grabbing one of his swinging legs with my free hand. The man in the seat in front peered angrily through the crack. Other passengers poked their heads in the aisle to check out the commotion my little boy was making.

'Is there anything I can help you with?' a friendly flight attendant leant over our seats with a bright white smile.

I glanced over at Max in his window seat. What had happened to my flirtatious little man? He stared angrily at the chair in front, not looking up at the gorgeous attendant at all. She tried to hand him an activity book with some colouring pencils. Still he did not look up. She placed them on his table.

'There you go, little man,' she said cheerfully. He did not even register her presence.

'Thank you,' I said, grateful to her for trying to help.

'No!' Max said, grabbing the little package and throwing it hard at the chair in front.

'Max! Very naughty!' I said, giving him a little smack on the leg.

He began wailing and screaming at the top of his lungs, and continued pretty much the whole way to Sydney. Usually chips or a lollypop would subdue him, but not this time. I just couldn't understand what had gotten into him and he just couldn't communicate to me what it was. This was a pattern that I would come to get used to over the years.

Eventually Max fell asleep just as we were descending into Sydney. Along with everyone else on the plane, I was grateful for the peace and quiet.

Mum picked us up from the airport. She would always wait right at the gate with a double pram, ready for the kids. I was so grateful to see her. Max was excited to see his Mimi too: we disembarked the plane and the flight from hell was forgotten as he ran into his Mimi's arms.

'There's just something special about the first grandchild,' Mum would say of Max. At the time, she didn't know that 'specialness' could be a burden as well as a blessing.

We stayed the night at Mum's house in Wahroonga and the following day I borrowed her car to drive into the city. Negotiating the busy Sydney traffic, I reminisced about the many times I had driven these roads as a teenager in my little Mazda 323. I giggled to myself, remembering how my friend Brad had helped me change the Mazda symbol on my 323 on the back of my car to read 'Madaz'. We thought that was hilarious, and so did many people driving behind me. Sometimes I missed that sense of irresponsibility. I had almost forgotten what it was like — only to have yourself to worry about. You don't realise how wonderful those carefree days are until they are well and truly gone.

Parking the car in the very familiar back lot of Fox Studios, I turned down Cyndi Lauper's 'Time after Time' on my mum's crappy CD player and fixed my makeup in the rear-vision mirror. For some reason I felt strangely confident.

In the studio I was met by one of the producer's personal assistants, who led me into the waiting area at the back of the warehouse where I could sit and wait for my audition. A few celebrities that I was vaguely familiar with walked past. I found it strange that I used to know everyone in the media, or at least recognise who they were. After taking a few years off to have kids, my head was full of the Wiggles and Thomas the Tank Engine. Now, if Anthony from The Wiggles walked by I would be excited!

After I had sat there for half an hour, going over my lyrics in my head, the personal assistant strode towards me. 'You're up, Chloe,' she said, waving me towards a soundproof door.

On the other side of the door was a large room with a couple of microphone stands in it. A slightly dishevelled-looking man with dreadlocks was standing there grinning as I entered.

'Hello, my name's Mark,' he said, shaking my hand politely.

'I'm Chloe,' I said, suddenly a little nervous.

'And this is everyone else.' He gestured to the far wall, which was made of glass. A gang of people were sitting there observing us. I recognised Chong Lim, who was famous from his role as musical director on the Australian version of *Dancing with the Stars* and of course his success in the music industry over the years.

I was asked to sing Cyndi Lauper's 'Time after Time' as well as 'Ain't No Mountain High Enough', which was a hit for Marvin Gaye and Tammi Terrell before Diana Ross took it to the top the charts. I thought I sounded pretty good. The judges seemed to be impressed with my performance as well, from what I could tell. They would let me know, they said.

Several weeks later I got the call I was waiting for.

'You got it, Chloe!' My manager Jane was ecstatic.

'When do I start?' I asked excitedly.

'Your lessons begin next week, then next month you will fly to Melbourne every weekend.'

This was going to be a logistical nightmare. Now I had to work out what I was going to do with the two kids while I was working and Mat was playing and training.

My vocal coach was a woman called Andy Gallagher, who had a quaint little apartment overlooking the valley and beach at Currumbin, a quiet pocket on the Gold Coast. A couple of times a week we spent an hour doing scales and working on my vocal technique.

Each celebrity on *It Takes Two* is assigned a professional mentor, all big names in the Australian music industry — Kate Ceberano, Ian Moss and Troy Cassar-Daley, to name a few. The first day of shooting was the 'big reveal' — me meeting my mentor. Mum flew up to Queensland to collect the kids and take them back to Sydney with her for a week or two. I flew to

Melbourne and met my mentor, the amazing David Campbell. I was elated that he would be my partner on the show, as he is incredibly talented and heaps of fun, too. The production crew filmed me walking into a café to meet David and then singing my first song to him against a backing track. I had chosen Moloko's 'Sing It Back', and I was nervous as hell. But David was stoked: I had pitch and rhythm, he told me, which was more than many contestants started with!

Over the next four weeks I flew back and forth, practising and performing with David. I was loving being back on television but it was a real juggling act with the kids. Was it also petrifying singing on national television? That's putting it mildly.

One weekend, I invited Dad to fly to Melbourne with Brodie to watch me perform. I thought this would be an ideal opportunity to make amends. Max had been staying with my mum in Sydney, so Dad and Brodie brought Max down with them. That way I could take him back to Queensland with me, rather than flying to Sydney to pick him up. Two men and a baby on a plane — it was a learning experience for all. Brodie demonstrated his latent parenting skills by changing a soiled nappy on the plane — as anyone who has had to do it will agree, that is never an easy task. Not bad going for a guy who didn't have children of his own.

I'll never forget rehearsing with David that day. We were singing Linda Ronstadt's 'Blue Bayou'. I stepped out on stage in a purple floor-length Wayne Cooper dress. The music began slowly.

'I feel so bad, I got a worried mind, I'm so lonesome all the time, since I left my baby behind on Blue Bayou,' I sang sombrely into the microphone. I opened my eyes as David began his verse and there were Dad, Brodie and Max. Dad's eyes were brimming with tears.

'I'll never be blue, my dreams come true on Blue Bayou.' We finished the song in harmony. Dad leapt to his feet, clapping and hollering while wiping tears from his eyes. Grant Denyer, the host, asked him why he was so emotional and he replied that he used to sing that song to me as a baby and it had meant a lot to him then.

I knew that the song was particularly special for him because it was one of his favourite songs. What I didn't know was that Dad was also emotional because of a secret he was keeping from me.

It was on this trip that Dad began noticing Max's severe developmental delays. He was afraid to say anything, though: we had only just made our peace and he didn't want to lose our relationship again. So he bided his time.

That night I was voted off the show, and thus ended one of the most terrifying but strength-giving experiences of my life. I had gone from housewife to TV star again, and it had frightened the life out of me and challenged me at one and the same time. I figured if I could sing on national television in front of more than a million viewers, I could do anything.

That theory was about to be tested beyond anything I could have imagined.

* * *

One day out of the blue I decided to call Jo and apologise. It was time we mended our relationship: we hadn't spoken for almost a year, though we had exchanged numerous vitriol-infused text messages.

Through firsthand experience, I had come to understand just how difficult it was being a stepmother and trying to please everybody. I understood the overwhelming sensation of being condemned by children who were not yours, yet because they were important to the man you loved, you would bend over backwards for them. I understood the feeling of complete helplessness when you tried your hardest, only to have it continually go unnoticed. I was beginning to understand how much Jo loved my dad and how over those many years she had stood up for him when he would not do it for himself. I saw a lot of similarities between Jo and I and between Mat and my dad. They had gone through what we were now going through, fifteen years later.

I was in a personal development seminar in Canberra when I had the overwhelming need to call Jo. Mat and I often went to these seminars to learn how to become better people and a stronger couple. We were in between sessions when I decided to duck out of the conference hall and call her. I hadn't even told Mat what I planned to do. Standing in an alcove with my hands shaking, I found her number in my phone. My finger hovered over the call button for at least thirty seconds, then I made the decision and pushed my finger down to call.

I listened to Jo's phone ring and as the seconds passed, my eyes filled with tears of relief. The simple fact that I had made the decision to apologise and to forgive was already mending every atom of hurt in my body, without me even having to talk to her. The burden I had been carrying with me for so many years had been lifted with this one split-second decision.

I credit this decision to my relationship with Jesus Christ. To this day I still can't quite explain it — and I won't try to here, because that is another story altogether. However, I constantly have revelations of ways my life can become better and how I can benefit other people's lives through Jesus' teachings. For many years I never imagined that I could become a believer. I had always thought I was too imperfect, too much of a sinner; but through a long journey of exploration, I came to understand that the basic principles of Christianity could help me in life, and that we were forgiven for our sins, but we were never called to be perfect.

'Hello, you've reached Joanne Maxwell of Chapel House. Sorry I couldn't take your call, but if you'd like to leave me a message I'll get right back to you.' I inhaled deeply.

'Hi Jo, this is Chloe.' My voice began to falter with emotion.

'I just wanted to call and say ... I am ... so sorry. I'm sorry for how I acted and I know you did the best you could for us as kids growing up. Call me when you can. Bye.' I hung up and made my way to the ladies' toilets, where I shut myself in a cubicle and let out the psychological torment and anguish I had been carrying around with me.

Baggage is a funny thing. The more you have of it, the heavier it becomes and the longer it takes you to reach your destination in life. Letting go through forgiveness is one of the greatest gifts you can give yourself. I believe it was Carrie Fisher who once said that 'resentment is like drinking poison and waiting for the other person to die'. Why we choose to hold onto bitterness and not to forgive is beyond me. I am convinced this is where cancer and other terminal diseases can come from. Let it go! Life is way too short.

Jo eventually called me back and we talked for an hour, crying together and apologising to each other. The bridge had been mended. Now, I can't imagine not having Dad and Jo in our life and in our children's lives. Max and Phoenix absolutely adore their nanna Jo and grandpa, as do Jack and Skyla.

13

Mat had always thought Max was not the same as other kids. He had tried to tell me on more than a dozen occasions, but I just refused to hear it. When Max was twelve months old, Mat became even more acutely aware of the differences. Perhaps coincidentally, it was just after Max had his measles, mumps and rubella (MMR) injection. After his vaccination, Max had quite a severe reaction: he vomited, he broke out in hives — but even though I was scared at the time, I assumed this was just what many babies go through. That's true, too, but it never occurred to me that this reaction might also be a forerunner of more serious and longer-term consequences.

It was a mid-week morning and Mat had just returned home from training. He usually had one session in the morning then a break before another session in the afternoon, so he would often come home to have lunch with us then head off to training again.

'Honey, I'm home.' I heard the garage door shut as I was cleaning in the kitchen.

'Hi, darling, how was training?' I said, rolling up the tea towel I had just been using and throwing it into the kitchen sink. Mat dropped his training bag and grabbed me in one of his strong embraces. He kissed me passionately on the lips.

'It was good but this is better,' he said cheekily.

He turned around to look for Max. While I had been cleaning the kitchen, Max had been playing so quietly with his trains in the lounge room that I had almost forgotten he was there.

'Hey, Maxi!' Mat called to him as he walked over towards him. Max didn't answer; he didn't even look up.

'Max.' Mat called his name louder. Still no response. He seemed to be extremely focused on pushing his Thomas train around the little wooden tracks.

Mat knelt down beside him. 'Where's my kiss from my big boy?' he asked, grabbing him affectionately. Max would not even look up from the Thomas train.

'What's wrong, mate?' Mat asked. He lifted Max's face up with one hand and tried desperately to get his little boy to look at him. Max would not look him in the eye. It seemed he would only look at his dad from out of the corner of each eye rather than front on. I thought he might have been playing a game, or perhaps he was just tired. I made many excuses for Max's behaviour; I was very good at it.

Mat gave up and walked back into the kitchen where I had

started to prepare dinner. He continued to look at Max, who had moved straight back to the wooden track and was pushing the train around the track in a rather eerie way, as though he were in a daze.

'Why isn't he kissing me anymore?' Max had always run to give his dad a big kiss when he got home from training. It did seem a little strange when I thought about it.

'And why can't he look at me?' Mat's voice was worried.

'He's probably just playing a silly game,' I said, shaking off the remarks but not wanting to get defensive and angry. Mat sat down on the kitchen stool and observed Max for a while.

Phoenix had woken up by this stage, so I went to check on her. I changed her nappy and brought her out into the kitchen to find Mat still staring worriedly at his son.

'Look, Daddy's here.' Phoenix's eyes lit up and a big smile exploded across her face as she looked at her daddy. Mat put out his arms to her and she did the same.

After they had hugged and Mat had kissed her all over her face, he turned to me again and said, 'There's something not right with Maxi. I'm worried about him.'

'He's fine,' I said with a tinge of anger as I went and picked Max up and cuddled him on the couch.

'He's fine.' I stroked his hair as he looked out to nothingness.

I was in denial.

* * *

One of the greatest inventions of the modern world, I truly believe, is online shopping. After discovering grocery shopping online, I never looked back.

One day I set out with Max and Phoenix to do a top-up shop of nappies, fresh food and frozen goods to fill the gaps in my online order. On the main road around the corner from our house was a vast shopping complex called the Q Super Centre, a strange cluster of buildings that just seemed to shoot up in the middle of nowhere. There were a lot of developing areas like this on the Gold Coast — concrete jungles surrounded by acres of vacant land.

I sat Max in the trolley and put Phoenix in the baby seat at the front of the trolley, her chubby little legs dangling as we proceeded into the supermarket. Max began to shift uncomfortably in his seat as we pushed through the swinging metal gate. As I stopped to grab some bananas in the fruit and vegetable section, Max started to look distressed. I tried to ignore him as I pushed the trolley through to the bread and cakes section. All of a sudden he began to scream uncontrollably, as though he was in pain. I began pushing the trolley faster down the aisles, my face turning crimson with embarrassment. I could feel everyone's eyes on us and I wanted to get this over and done with as quickly as possible. I glanced down at Phoenix: she seemed to be having a great time, smiling at everyone and enjoying a fun ride in the trolley.

'How can the two of them be having such completely different experiences right now?' I puzzled to myself.

It was as though with every new aisle the experience became even more overwhelming for Max.

'You be a good boy and you can have some chippies,' I cajoled, in the hope that a bribe would calm him down. He did love his chips. But this time he took no notice of me whatsoever, instead looking from left to right with a look I could only label as straight-up fear. He was afraid of something — but what?

By the time we finally reached the checkout, his screams had not ceased. I had opened chips, chocolates, drinks — anything I thought could possibly calm him down was useless. The opened packages were piled in my hands for fear of him spilling their contents all over our groceries in his fit of hysteria.

In the queue ahead of us was a slightly older mother with three children. The two younger kids were boys and would have been a similar age to Max and Phoenix, and the third was a little girl who looked around five. The youngest was in a BabyBjörn attached to his mum's chest, the other boy was in the baby seat of the trolley. The little girl was helping her mum unload the groceries for scanning, all the while silently observing Max as though he was some sort of oddity.

The checkout operator turned a sympathetic eye to us as she scanned the woman's groceries. Once there was room on the conveyor belt I quickly began to unload my own goods, pretending that there was nothing out of the ordinary happening.

Max's screams had reached a critical level when I decided I had a choice to make. I had to say or do something. Everyone in the whole bloody shopping centre was staring at us as though we were lepers. 'Am I going to be one of those cranky stressed-out mums that shouts incessantly at their kids in public areas, or can I somehow make light of the situation?' I asked myself. All hell might be breaking loose around me but I have the choice, I can decide how I will react, I told myself. And decide I did.

'I will never take my sister's kids shopping ever again!' I blurted while giving the checkout operator a cheeky wink and my credit card.

The mother of the three perfectly behaved kids rolled her eyes and nodded in agreement as she walked her trolley and perfect kids out the door.

'Huh! Chloe, one, ridiculously competent mother of three perfect kids, zero!' I muttered under my breath.

'Hi, Chloe; hello, Max; hi, Phoenix,' the checkout lady said. 'Nice photo of the whole family on page three of the *Bulletin*.' She pointed at a pile of local papers next to the stack of grocery baskets.

I always forgot how many people on the Gold Coast knew who Mat was and consequently knew all about us and our business. Oh well. I still felt victorious!

Thank goodness perfect mum of three was out of earshot, I thought as I smiled and nodded — not that she would have heard much over the constant din of Max's discontent.

That was the last time Max would enter a grocery store for a very long time.

14

Why should those lovers that no lovers miss
Dream, until God burn Nature with a kiss?

— W.B. Yeats, 'The Man who Dreamed of Faeryland'

When Mat and I got married in October 2008, we didn't fit the usual bridal party template. Mat had been married once before and had two children from that marriage, and together we had two more children.

I had never really pictured myself having the standard white wedding, anyway — I wanted something different, and the traditional approach didn't seem to fit us. So for starters, I chose a beautiful floor-length gown in a rich emerald-green (my favourite colour) as my wedding dress — far from your typical bridal outfit.

It had been a year since Phoenix was born and I was determined to get back in shape, so I set to work training almost every day. I had a personal trainer for some sessions and on the other days I would be at the gym doing RPM or Pump classes.

For several years my body had been owned by my children, from carrying them in the womb to feeding them. It felt great to have control of my body again.

By the time our wedding weekend came around I had lost ten kilograms. All of my baby fat had disappeared and then some — I was ecstatic! Thank God, because I had a figure-hugging Alex Perry gown I needed to squeeze into.

We decided to hold our wedding at the Hyatt in Sanctuary Cove on the Gold Coast in Queensland. We wanted to make it a massive celebration, with events for our guests across the entire weekend. Mat and I were pretty easygoing; all we wanted was for our guests to have an absolute ball.

We had engaged the Classic Events Company to plan the wedding for us. They were responsible for organising some pretty impressive events on the Gold Coast. The owner, Phil Harte, had assured us they would take care of everything — festivities, food, security, the lot. We had a deal in place with *OK* magazine, which meant that they would cover the wedding costs in return for exclusive rights to publish our wedding photos in their magazine.

As our guests checked in to the hotel on the Friday, they received a lanyard detailing the events for the weekend. To kick off the festivities, we had arranged for our immediate family to join us for dinner at the restaurant downstairs. It would be one of the very few times that my dad and Jo had been in the same room as my mum and Ross since Mum and Dad divorced, all those years ago. I was incredibly nervous about how they would interact.

The restaurant was a cosy place with an enormous fireplace oven. There were around twenty of us in our group. When everyone was seated, Mat and I decided to say a few words. I stood there looking at my two families, who had fought for two decades over the collapse of a marriage. Sitting there together, there was no trace of the hostility that had reigned for so long. They were together again, unified for the purpose of a new life — a life together for Mat and me.

I looked at my mum and dad clinking glasses in celebration and my heart was filled with joy. As a child all I had ever wanted was for them to get along. I knew they had their differences, but they would always be my parents. My mum and my dad, two of the most important people in my life. It meant the world to me, to see them getting along after so many years.

The dinner was happily uneventful. Indeed, it seemed as though Mum and Dad were really beginning to enjoy themselves in each other's company. I didn't know it then, but it was an important first step towards Mum and Dad coming together to help me in my time of need.

The next morning, our close friends and family members were escorted to the helipad and given a surprise helicopter ride along the coastline. Many guests were ecstatic to see wild dolphins in the ocean below them.

That evening we held a welcome cocktail party down by the lagoon. Mat and I got there early to greet everyone as they walked in.

'Darling, I've got some exciting news.' Mat pulled me aside just after we had greeted a large group of people.

'What's that?' I asked, wondering how this weekend could get any better.

'Dave Faulkner is going to sing for us tonight,' he said with his trademark sexy grin.

'Oh my gosh,' I exclaimed. Dave is the lead singer of the iconic Australian rock band, Hoodoo Gurus; he had been a friend of Mat's for a very long time, so he was at the wedding as our guest.

The crowd of about a hundred and eighty people erupted into applause as the famous Australian singer took his position centre stage with his guitar. He played classics like 'What's my Scene?', 'Bittersweet' and 'Miss Freelove '69'. It was a moment in time.

When the welcome party came to an end, the boys were taken to watch the Gold Coast Blaze basketball team in VIP seating as a buck's night treat. Why my husband decided to have his buck's night the evening before our wedding day I will never know. At least he made it, though, and didn't end up tied naked to a flagpole somewhere in Surfers Paradise.

Luckily, the wedding was not until the following evening, which gave everyone the chance to recover and regroup after the night before. I had a brunch organised for the ladies while the men went to play golf. My mum had decided not to come; instead she took the kids off my hands. Max had been quite unsettled through the celebrations, so she would have her work cut out for her. I was a little disappointed: I really wanted Mum there and I didn't mind if the kids were there too. But she was determined that that was what she would do, so I let her be.

The brunch was held on the immaculate lawn opposite our room. Tables were laid with white tablecloths and filled with a gorgeous spread of cakes, tea, coffee, orange juice and champagne. I was having a really pleasant morning when Mum wheeled Max up to see how we were doing. She puffed the fringe off her forehead, clearly stressed.

'How's it going?' she asked, looking around at everyone having a good time.

'Really good, Mum. Why don't you just hang out? Maxi can be here, it's OK,' I said, really wanting to spend some time with her. She was the mother of the bride after all.

'No, I'm going to take him upstairs for a sleep. Grandma has just taken Phoenix upstairs.'

Sometimes Mum would say one thing but I could see that she meant something else. She was clearly unhappy being with the kids and not being part of the brunch. I know she just wanted me to enjoy myself without the stress of the kids, but I think I was more stressed watching her deal with them and not enjoying herself.

'I'll be up at 2 to iron your dress,' she said as she turned and wheeled Max away up the path. I exhaled. 'OK,' I said, and turned to chat with my sister.

Once the brunch was over I headed up to my room to begin the lengthy hair and makeup process with all of my bridesmaids

— four in total, including my sister. Max was the ring bearer and Skyla and Phoenix were the flower girls. Maxi looked splendid in black pants and a little bow tie over a white shirt; Phoenix and Skyla wore gorgeous matching white dresses.

Once we were all made up, a golf buggy came to collect us from the hotel and drive us down to the lagoon for the photo session. The photographer wanted to take some shots of us standing and sitting on rocks and posing by the pool. I was to be the first one photographed, so she directed me into the foliage next to the lagoon. I was trying to step carefully when suddenly I felt my dress pulling. Looking down, I saw that I had put my heel straight through my gown. 'Oh no. I haven't even walked down the aisle in it yet,' I squeaked, understanding in that moment how brides could become bridezillas. In the background, Max was screaming; a lot of our wedding photos feature Max looking red in the face from crying.

Next a shriek comes from Dad. Turning to see what the problem was, I saw him holding Phoenix with a look of disgust on his face. She had soiled her nappy and I believe it had leaked onto his hand.

'Let's get this over and done with,' I snapped at the photographer. It was all I could do not to let every obscenity known to man come out of my mouth right then.

After the photos were finished, my bridesmaid Melissa took Phoenix and changed her on the floor of the penthouse in the Hyatt. Any other time it would have been hilarious, watching her kneeling in her beautiful gown and wrestling to extract an outrageously dirty nappy from under a cute little flower girl's dress.

We finally got ourselves straightened out, then it was time to head down to the hotel lobby. From there I would walk down the sandstone steps and past a beautiful water feature to where my husband-to-be would be waiting.

Dad and I hovered nervously, peering out the windows at the assembled guests below. The bridesmaids were already positioned at the top of the stairs behind the door, just out of sight.

'I'm so proud of you, darling.' Dad's blue eyes were moist with tears as he put his arms around me.

'Thanks, Dad,' I said, as the first sounds of the wedding drifted in through the windows. I had organised for three women to sing an a cappella version of Soul II Soul's song 'Back to Life' as I walked down the aisle. I heard them hit the first note.

First out was Skyla holding Phoenix. I watched Skyla navigate the stairs. Everyone seemed to be holding their breath, hoping she wouldn't drop her little sister. Mat's eyes lit up when he saw his two daughters coming down the stairs towards him.

Next were the bridesmaids: one by one they came out, looking elegant in different styles of black dresses. 'It's time,' Phil whispered to us and we followed him down to the door. Then his walkie-talkie buzzed urgently: there was an intruder. Phil placed his hand in front of me to prevent me from walking out and made a call to security. Several security guards ran through the assembled wedding guests and a rogue cameraman was apprehended.

'OK, you're safe to go,' Phil said and Dad and I stepped out onto the top step. A light wind picked up my emerald-green gown as I clutched one side of it to walk down the stairs. The tempo of the music had picked up; Dad and I were so excited we almost ran to the altar.

My eyes came to rest on Mat. He looked so incredibly handsome that day, I thought I would melt. The closer I got the more I saw the emotion etched in his face, until our hands touched and my dad let his daughter go.

After our vows, fireworks erupted. Max loved those — he wasn't scared by the noise and lights at all. We gathered the other kids up in our arms; we were all now joined as one. I had married those children just as much as their dad and I intended to honour that for the rest of my life.

15

Now as at all times I can see in the mind's eye,
In their stiff, painted clothes, the pale unsatisfied ones …

— W.B. Yeats, 'The Magi'

Max's second Christmas was spent in Woy Woy, on the Central Coast of New South Wales, with my dad's family. We made the trek down with all four kids in tow. Dad and Jo had rented a house right on the bay for all of us to stay in. It was nice and close to where Dad's other relatives were staying, but I worried all the time about the little ones being so close to the water. Max was obsessed with water, dripping taps in particular. Often I would call out to him and get no answer, then walk around the side of the house to find him watching the tap — drip, drip, drip — and plugging it with his finger every few drips.

I was constantly trying to cover for Max that Christmas. If anyone directed any questions at him, I would answer them for him every time. I tried to stick him in front of a DVD as much as possible so his strangeness wouldn't be as noticeable.

Max always seemed to have a glazed look in his eyes, whereas his cousin Cooper, who was around the same age, engaged with everyone. He would tell stories, he would laugh; he had a very impressive knowledge of cows and cowboys and guns. Max spoke, but it was another language. 'Gobbledygook', I called it. It didn't make sense and it was never really directed at anyone, as Max wasn't in the habit of looking people in the eye. I could see a big difference in development between Max and Cooper and it frightened me.

One night when we were all sitting around the campfire, Dad pulled Mat and me aside.

'I wanted to speak to you both about Max.' I gulped and directed my attention to the campfire shadows licking at the roots of the surrounding trees. I imagined the surrounding bush suddenly engulfed in flames and my relatives running for the water in terror.

'I have some serious concerns about his development.' The flames began to lick at my heels and dance up my legs; my face turned the colour of fire. I turned and looked at Mat. His face was hidden in darkness so I couldn't see his expression. I turned slowly back to this devil in my father's clothing.

'I've done some research and I believe he may be autistic.' Suddenly my whole body was on fire with rage; the heat was unbearable.

'What are you talking about?' I shouted from the depths of flaming darkness. 'There is nothing wrong with my little boy!

Why are you saying this? Because of Cooper, because he can talk better than Max? He's four months older that's all — he … he …' My larynx had swollen as though I was being overcome by smoke fumes.

I felt Mat's strong arms embrace me, holding my arms down to prevent me from flailing wildly at my father. I wanted to hurt him. I wanted him to feel the pain I was feeling. My daddy was hurting me, so much. I don't know what words came out of my mouth then, but they were hateful and hurtful.

Tears began to put out the fire in my face as I looked at my dad, his blue eyes glistening with sadness in the dark. Jo stood next to him, afraid to look at me. Her eyes were fixed on the ground and streaming with tears. The angry words spurting from my mouth subsided as Mat spun me around to look at him. His face was contorted with a sadness I had only ever witnessed once before, when he had just seen his father's body in a stairwell in Cronulla.

'I agree with your dad, darling,' Mat said hoarsely. 'Max isn't the same as other kids, Chloe, I've felt that for a while, but every time I've tried to talk to you about it you've gotten angry and shut me down.' I could feel the pain running through his strong tattooed arms. That strength couldn't help him with this fight.

My bottom lip was quivering uncontrollably.

'We can't keep ignoring this!' Mat broke down sobbing and so did I, as we both came to the realisation that we — or rather, I — had been in denial all this time.

As soon as we got back to Queensland I booked an appointment with a paediatrician and I began to read. Dad and Jo had given me the *Australian Autism Handbook* by Seana Smith and Benison O'Reilly which I found invaluable. I scoured the internet for any information I could find on autism. I knew very little about it. All I knew was taken from watching Dustin Hoffman's performance in the movie *Rain Man*, and I did not think that was Max.

Even though I certainly didn't want to concede that Max might be autistic, even I had to admit that he was a difficult child. He was two and a half now, and he had the most incredibly violent tantrums. Having no other example to go by, I thought this was standard behaviour for the terrible twos. And being pretty strong-willed myself, I just thought that he took after me.

He would not answer to his name, no matter how much I shouted at him. He wouldn't even turn around and look at me — it was as if he was looking out into another dimension. I wanted to rule out all the other possibilities before I would consider that he might have autism, so we decided to have his hearing checked. I made an appointment to go and see a hearing specialist. Mat would be at training, so I would have to take him on my own.

At the hearing specialist's Max was more interested in playing with the sliding door and watching it glide back and forth over and over again than he was in going into the little room with the toys. His screams were piercing as the specialist and I tried to drag him away from his beloved sliding door. We managed to get him into the little dark room with much protesting on his behalf. From what the specialist could gather from her limited scrutiny of a howling Max, his hearing was fine.

'He has perfect hearing in at least one ear,' she told me as I signed the Medicare form. My head began to reel. I had been hoping it would be a hearing problem that grommets would fix. I had a girlfriend who had found out that her son's ear canals hadn't opened properly and he was partially deaf because of it. She said he got grommets and he was one hundred per cent now. That had given me so much hope and now that hope was gone.

When February came round I spent several days in bed, not wanting to leave the house. The weight of my little angel's condition lay heavily on my shoulders as I debated whether I had caused it somehow. 'What did I do wrong? What should I have done differently?' I played the blame game with myself for several days, unable to move from my cocoon.

I spent the next few days reading stories of children with autism and realised that Max had too many similarities to these other cases for him not to be in the same category. My heart felt heavy with loss, but at the same time I told myself that my little boy was still here — he wasn't dead, and he was still my little boy.

After reading and teetering on the brink of depression for three days I finally decided it was time to tell my family. I didn't have a diagnosis in writing yet, but I knew.

I rang my mum and just came out with it. No beating around the bush. I had already gone through all of the different emotions — anger, blame, fear, devastation and a feeling of loss, and now I was ready to fight! And fight I did.

'Hi, Mum.' I was short with her, angry. 'I just called to tell you that Max is autistic. I thought you should know.' Silence on the other end of the phone.

'How do you know?' Her voice was small, faraway.

'I just do. I don't really want to talk about it much more today. I'm going to go now.' And with that I hung up the phone.

Less than half an hour passed and my phone started ringing.

'I'm so sorry, Chloe, we just heard the news.' One by one my brother, my sister and a bunch of other relatives called. Mum had obviously phoned everyone to pass on the news. How infuriating!

'Sorry for what? My boy is not dead!' I was livid.

I called Mum back and absolutely ripped into her. I just couldn't believe she could get off the phone from me after I said I didn't want to talk about it anymore, and immediately start calling everyone. How could she be so insensitive? I know she meant well, but that sort of news is something I should have shared with them myself when I was ready.

'How dare you go and tell everyone!' I screamed into the receiver at her, my hands shaking with rage. 'I don't want anyone feeling sorry for him or me. He isn't dead, you know!' My entire body began convulsing.

'You're an alien, Chloe!' She screamed back. 'I can't even talk to you anymore, I have to walk on eggshells!' I could almost taste the vitriol in her voice. Who was this woman?

'My son is autistic, Mum, I am trying to come to terms with that!' I hung up the phone.

I began getting inundated with calls from various relatives. One asked if I had dropped Max on his head as a baby, another blamed Jack for spinning him around too much or being too rough with him. Others blamed my work, claiming I wasn't around enough (I was with him every day!) or that he watched too much television. I wondered how they could keep such good tabs on us from a thousand kilometres away. You name it, they blamed it.

Until they are in a situation where they need to find out more, most people just don't know what autism is. They don't know that it's not caused by spinning kids around, or watching too much television, or 'refrigerator mums' who are emotionally distant from their children. Usually the people who know most are mothers whose own children have an ASD — those mothers know more about the condition than many GPs.

But at this point, I wasn't coping with my relatives' ignorance at all well. The one time I needed emotional support from my family more than ever, and this is what I got. With every cutting comment I boiled on the inside. Why were they attacking me? Yes, I was defensive, but why shouldn't I be? This was my issue — this was my son, for heaven's sake!

I guess I had always been the irresponsible one growing up. I was the party girl, the one who burnt plastic trays in the oven thinking they were ovenproof, the one who was out clubbing from the age of sixteen, the one who no-one ever thought would have kids that would actually survive. At the time I was probably thinking too much about myself and not enough about what I was doing. My mother once told me she had a nightmare about me dropping off my baby to her in a shoebox. Any time I had joked, 'Mum, I've got something to tell you — I'm pregnant,' she would reply, 'You're leaving home,' giving me the distinct impression that she didn't think me capable of looking after a child. At that particular time she was probably right. But now I was dealing with a stereotype left over from my childhood as well as with my son's condition.

Isn't it amazing when you grow up but your family still thinks of you as a child?

One of the things I'd always wanted more than anything was to be a mother. Not only that, I wanted to be the best mother. I'm the type of person that wants to be the best at everything that I do, and I guess I get upset when I'm not. I just adore my family: they come first in everything that I do, in any decisions I make. There's a book called *The Five Love Languages* that describes the different ways people show their love. My love language is 'acts of service'. I clean the house, I cook — I love doing all those domestic things. From the minute I get up in the morning, I'm doing things for my family. And the minute I go to bed, I'm already thinking about how I can do, be or have more for them the next day.

Some days I feel as though I am the perfect mother, but not every day. I can get caught up in cleaning the house and baking — I love to have a spotless house and good food on the table — but I think kids want time more than anything else. They probably won't remember the banana bread I made from scratch on one of my 'perfect' days, but they will definitely remember me being at the park with them, getting on the pedal car and pushing them on the swing. Those are the memories that stay with children.

Most of all, I didn't want my kids to go through what I went through as a child — the divided family, the tug of war between parents. More than anything I wanted to create the dream family, because I didn't feel that I had that when I was growing up.

This would have to have been one of the lowest points in my life. My husband and I had each other and that was it. I had always turned to Mum in times of need, but her response to me criticising her was to attack me for a whole bunch of things I had done wrong in the past that were totally irrelevant to the current situation.

Those closest to you can cause so much more pain than complete strangers. Horrible emails bounced back and forth as I tried to defend myself, my way of parenting and my need to have an active role in providing for my family financially. In the heat of the moment, words were said that were absolutely devastating at the time. I still bear scars from them, and I'm sure others do too.

Deep down I knew I was a good mother to my kids, but I was finding it hard enough to deal with the realisation that my son had autism, let alone having family members persecute me for things they felt I had done to make my son be this way. I can see now they were just going through the stages of anger and blame that I had experienced myself. Since then they have shown remorse for how they acted, but at the time I felt incredibly hurt and completely alone.

One of Mat's teammates at the Titans was a lovely guy called Mark Minichiello. Mark and his wife Milena have always been deeply committed to learning more about health and wellbeing. Milena was a radiotherapist, which may have been one of the reasons they were so dedicated to wellness. When you are seeing cancer patients almost every day, I can imagine it would be a recurring wake-up call.

One night we were at the Titanium Bar in Surfers Paradise for a post-match function. I was thinking about Max a lot, so I wasn't really my usual bubbly self that night. Milena noticed.

'What's up, Chloe, are you OK?' she asked, plonking herself down in the chair next to me.

'Not really,' I answered, quite glad someone was prepared to hear my woes. 'I think Max might be autistic,' I said, blinking tears from my eyes.

'Oh, honey, I've read a lot of books on that subject,' she said, surprising me.

I opened up to Milena that night. I told her my fears and how frightened I was of what lay ahead. She in turn told me about her fear that she would have a child with that same condition. There was no family history of it, but as a health professional she was more aware than most people of the many things that can go wrong for children. (She is actually now pregnant with her first child as I write this chapter.) She had some exposure to autism and become intrigued by it, so she had done extensive research on the subject. It was Milena who gave me some of the first books I read on autism back then, including Jenny McCarthy's *Louder Than Words*. I devoured that book in one day, reading it through my tears.

McCarthy's child seemed to me to have much more severe symptoms than Max. According to her book he suffered from constant fits. She writes about one morning when there was no sound coming from his bedroom. She went to check on him and he was convulsing savagely in his bed with the whites of his eyes showing. That was the first indication that there was something wrong with her little boy.

I thank the Lord I have never experienced that with Maxi and hope I never will. It is, however, very common for autistic children to develop epilepsy later in life, so I guess we will just have to cross that bridge if we come to it.

Jenny McCarthy strongly believes that the measles, mumps and rubella (MMR) vaccine caused her son's decline. In the US, where Jenny lives, as well as in Australia, this injection is administered to children at the age of twelve months as a standard procedure. She also believes that with a gluten- and casein-free diet, her son became more lucid.

I have since read conflicting studies on the MMR side of things. Mat is quite convinced that at the very least, such a powerful shot containing so many different vaccines must surely affect each child differently, depending on their genetic makeup. Certainly the pharmaceutical industry (and consequently the government) makes a vast amount of money out of vaccines, so there are some compelling reasons for them to claim that there is no causal link between immunisations and autism. But it's a very controversial area still and it's hard to know what to believe: experts such as the World Health Organisation and the American Academy of Paediatrics believe there is no link between this immunisation and autism. In fact, there was a clinical trial in Japan in which immunisation stopped and the statistics show an increase in autism. There have also not been any real clinical trials that can prove a change of diet can help; however, this was something I wanted to try, at least.

As soon as I finished reading Jenny McCarthy's book I went through our pantry and threw out anything that contained gluten (a protein found in most cereals and bread) or casein (a protein found in milk). Extreme, I know, but this was my son's life we were talking about.

Luckily my local supermarket had a whole aisle dedicated to gluten- and casein-free foods, as do most of the big chain supermarkets these days. I could not believe how many things contained these ingredients: wheat and milk is used in pretty much everything that we eat.

I spent a small fortune and restocked our pantry with gluten- and casein-free foods from top to bottom. I was so incredibly strict with this diet that the whole family was on it for a while. Mat ended up losing too much weight, though, and had to go back to regular food. He couldn't risk the weight loss during football season. It made it all the more difficult when one of us was back on normal food. If Mat was cooking his gluten-filled toast, he was assigned one side of the toaster and the gluten-free bread went in the other. Mat's sister Melanie had had significant success with excluding these products from her son Cooper's diet; Cooper has Down's syndrome. It seemed that developmental delays for Down's syndrome kids could also be improved with dietary changes. Mel told me that if Max ingested even the smallest amount of gluten, all our efforts would be in vain. He may as well just be eating an unrestricted diet. So I became the Toaster Cop.

I also believe that tragic events during pregnancy can have a hand in babies being born different. There have been a few scientific studies along these lines, showing how stressful life events experienced by pregnant women can disrupt brain development in unborn babies.[1] Cooper had been born shortly after Mat and Melanie's mother Carol lost her long and painful battle with breast cancer. He wasn't diagnosed in the womb: Mel even had the nuchal translucency test to determine if Down's syndrome was present and it came up negative. It wasn't until Cooper was well into the world that his parents found out he had Down's syndrome.

More recently research suggests that children with autism are born with too many brain cells in a key area of the brain. It all starts in the womb, when the part of the brain that controls language and communication, as well as mood, attention and social ability, simply grows too fast.[2]

Brain development I couldn't control: diet I could, and did. After about a month of diet restrictions we went to see the paediatrician. In the waiting room there was a caged area with an assortment of toys for kids to play with. It reminded me of a kiddy prison: parents drop them in there and they can't escape. I dropped Max into his usual cellblock. He always obsessed over the Thomas the Tank Engine that was one of the many toys scattered there for inmates. His fascination with trains was completely over the top at the best of times, another indicator he may be on the spectrum. I know now that autistic kids are obsessively drawn to trains, especially Thomas, for some unknown reason. At least Thomas served to keep Max mildly amused while we waited to see the doctor. He calmly turned its little wheels over and over, watching them ever so closely.

'Max Rogers,' the secretary called. Now came the big challenge: leaving the train behind to go into the doctor's office. The screams and kicking would not subside, I knew, even when we were inside the doctor's office surrounded by thousands more toys specifically there to calm children and keep them occupied whilst the doctor addresses the parent. I grabbed the little train and put it in Max's hand. I marched past the receptionist with the little train embedded in Max's little hand, hidden beneath the hem of my loose-fitting top. Bugger if I'm going to deal with a tantrum like that when I know what will ease the pain. That train was coming with us.

In the office the doctor began with his usual line of questioning. 'How's little Max going?' he enquired, hardly looking up from his computer screen.

'Actually, he's been OK — his tantrums are still there but I've put him on a gluten- and casein-free diet and that seems to have made a slight difference. I can't tell for sure though,' I said imploringly, seeking some sort of approval in his eyes. Instead he sniggered. Not a polite laugh, but the kind that makes you feel as though everyone else thinks you're a fool.

'I wouldn't get too caught up in all of that stuff.' At his words I felt as though I had shrunk to the size of a small child. My face went bright red with anger; I could feel the heat rising on my cheeks.

'Was he being condescending to me right now?' I asked myself. Aloud, I asked, 'Really?' my voice breaking slightly with rage.

'I can do some blood tests if you want to test to see if he has an intolerance to those things, but it's not likely,' the doctor said with a decidedly I-know-better-than-you tone in his voice.

'Yes, please,' I said, my stomach burning with contempt. My cheeks were fatigued by the effort of holding on to the fake smile I had painted on.

'Why must everybody treat me like I should know everything, or like I know nothing? I'm trying my best here!' I thought, not knowing whether to scream or cry.

'How long have you had him on the diet for? He needs to have been consuming gluten and casein for at least a month for my tests to be effective.' He studied his notes through thick spectacles.

'A month,' I answered, my heart sinking.

'Well, you're going to need to put him back on normal food for a month before I can do any blood tests.'

I don't know if it was intentional on the doctor's part but I felt like I was back at school, being spoken to like a child. Either that or I just felt downright ridiculous for having gone to such extreme lengths without consulting with a doctor first.

'OK, so I'll take him off his diet and we will have tests in a month, then we'll be back for the results after that.' Great, more waiting. I was so sick of not having clarity, not having a strong sense that we were on the right path for my little man.

I left the doctor's office and stopped at the reception desk to make yet another appointment for a month's time. I had to pry Thomas from Max's fingers so I could put the toy back in the kiddy jail. Max did not want to leave that Thomas behind, so he decided this was the time he should have a complete meltdown. He screamed and kicked me and tried to gouge my face with his nails in front of a whole waiting room filled with people. His face had contempt written all over it. One mother, whose two children had sat ever so politely and quietly sifting through magazines, pulled her kids toward her in an attempt to protect them from this out-of-control child having a meltdown over a toy train.

'I could reach her with my foot from here, kick her right in her cat's-bum mouth!' I indulged myself with that fantasy as I wrestled Max out the door. His screams echoed through the car park, bouncing and reverberating off every wall as though there was more than one of him. We finally got to the car and despite his violent writhing I managed to buckle my little boy into his seat. I got into the driver's seat and broke down into uncontrollable sobbing. My tears of defeat glistened on the steering wheel. I looked up into the rear-view mirror and studied the scratches on my jaw and cheek. He had actually drawn blood with the one on my cheek.

It feels terrible for your son to want to hurt you so badly that you bleed, and to look into his beautiful eyes and see nothing but hatred. What mother could deal with that? Not me, that's for sure.

I felt like we were getting nowhere. Every time I thought I was moving forward, I was hurtled backwards even faster. I loved my son, but I was no longer sure whether I was the right mother for this job.

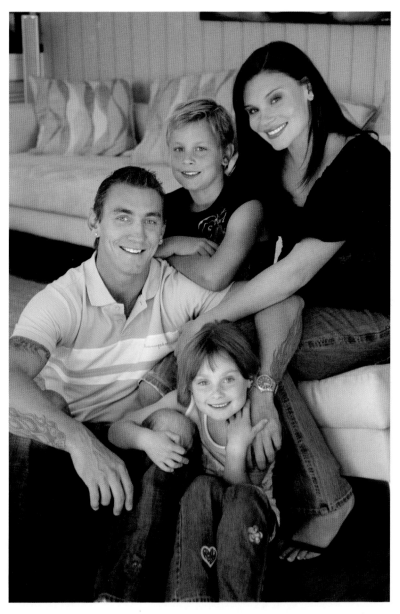

At our home in Cronulla — Mat, Jack, Skyla and me, when I was pregnant with Max. After his father Steve's death, Cronulla held sad memories so Mat jumped at the chance to make a fresh start and move to Queensland to play for the Gold Coast Titans in 2005.

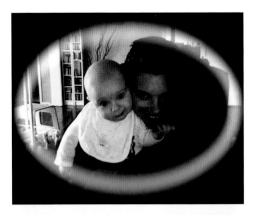

Max was about 2 months old here. He smiled at the camera just like any other baby would.

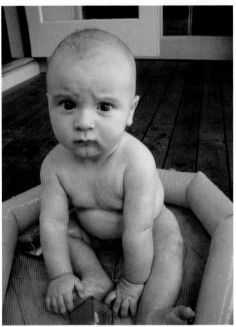

Max at 3 months old. He was my first child and I had a hard time accepting the fact that he had Autism Spectrum Disorder.

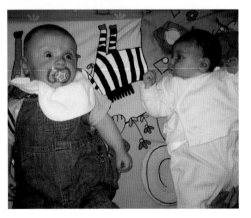

Max and his cousin Eden. Eden was a few months younger than Max. They were both still too young to see any difference in their development here, but later on Eden would well surpass Max.

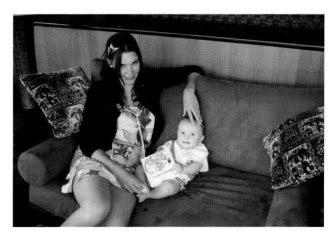

Max and me at the Sheraton Mirage on the Gold Coast. I loved reading to Max. My mum, whom the kids call 'Mimmi' had bought him this book called *Mimmi's Toes*.

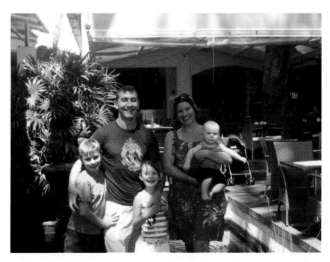

Jack, Mat, Skyla, me and Max on a holiday in Port Douglas. In those early years, the times when we were all together were extremely precious.

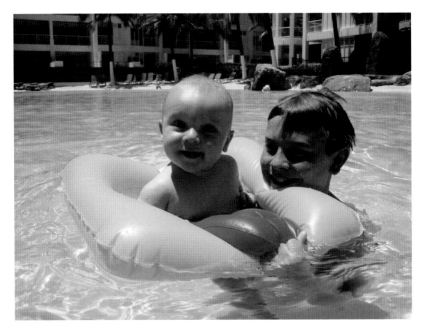

Jack and Max in the pool on our Port Douglas holiday. Max loved
the water then – still does – and used to smile all the time.

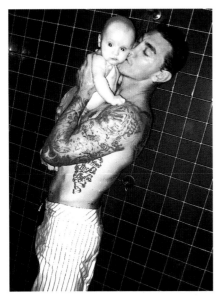

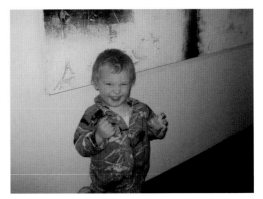

Max used to giggle and show his
muscles all the time, but after he
turned one, he stopped doing it.
It was one of the first signs that
something was wrong.

Mat and Max having a shower
together. Mat loves kids and
would have been quite happy for
me to have hundreds of them!

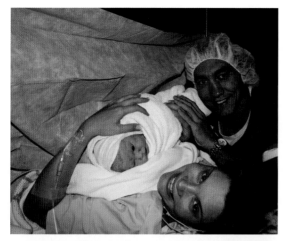

No matter what anyone tells you, nothing prepares you for holding your baby for the first time. Mat, myself and baby Phoenix at the hospital on 19 September 2007.

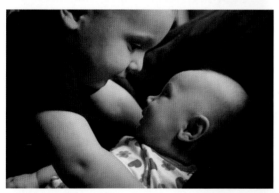

When Phoenix came along there was a massive shift in Max's personality and temperament. He has always loved babies and still smiles at them to this day.

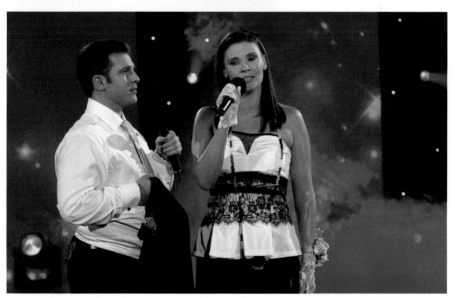

David Campbell and I on *It Takes Two*. Flying to Melbourne every week was a logistical nightmare with four kids and Mat training six days a week, but it reminded me that as well as being a mother, I had other talents and a career. (Courtesy of Channel 7.)

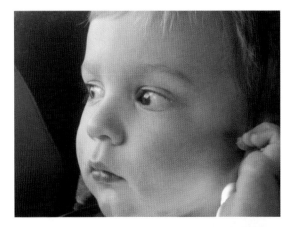

Max and his trademark 'staring-into-space' look. This was when he began to go backwards developmentally. We just had no idea why yet, or how to help him.

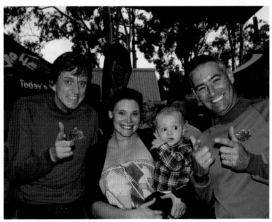

Working for a local radio show — SeaFM on the Gold Coast — came with a few perks. Max loved The Wiggles and got a chance to meet them one day. Not sure he was as excited as I was!

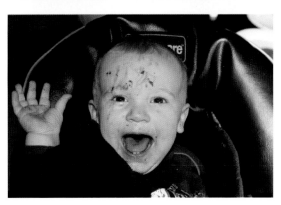

Max covered in Vegemite in his high chair. Sometimes when he was having a meltdown I would try to distract him with food — it didn't always work though!

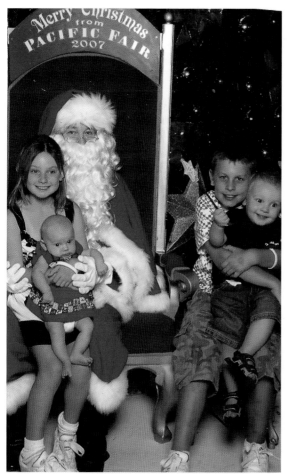

My own Christmas miracle – all four children with Santa. It was a real struggle to get Max to smile and stay put – you can see just how tight Jack had to hold him. Santa's helper gave him a toy to keep him occupied.

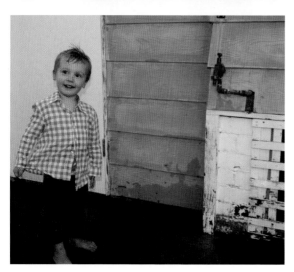

Max at Woy Woy when we spent Christmas with Dad and Jo. He had an obsession with water and couldn't stop watching the tap drip – it was this obsession that concerned Dad and made him think Max might have autism.

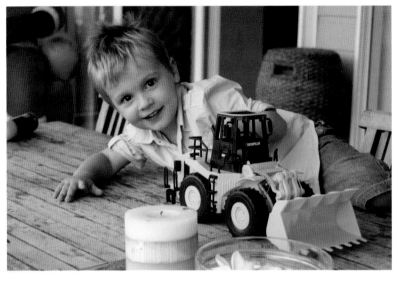

Look at that sweet little unsuspecting face!

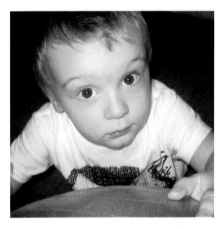

Max at our home in Clear Island Waters. His beautiful big brown eyes would often look right through you, not acknowledging you even if you greeted him or asked him a question.

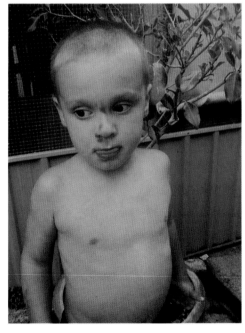

It is the worst feeling in the world to see your child bleed. Our hopes of a peaceful Christmas at Mat's Aunt Teresa's were dashed when Max fell over while playing with a remote-controlled truck. He wasn't at all fazed by the blood.

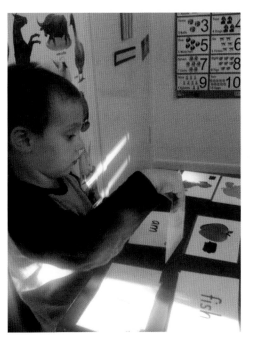

Max during therapy at Little Souls Taking Big Steps. Doing simple tasks over and over again, like matching words with symbols, was critical to his development. Little Souls Taking Big Steps inspired Mat and me to start our own charity so that parents of autistic children could afford the best treatment possible.

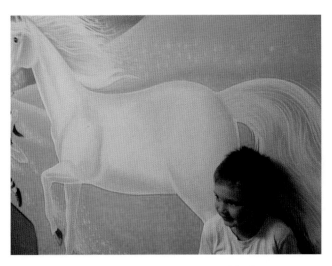

Max at a friend's birthday party at 2bkids in Burleigh Heads. He loves unicorns and spent more time with this wall than running around. Many children with ASD don't get to experience the simple pleasures of going to a friend's birthday party because their parents fear they might 'cause a scene'.

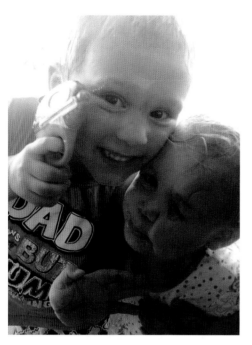

Max and Phoenix peeping through our glass door at Mermaid Beach in 2010. Max was making great progress with his therapy and she really helped that by reinforcing what he'd learnt.

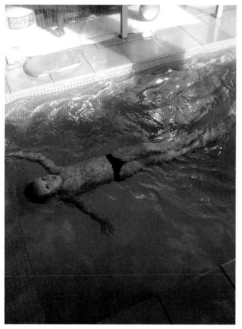

Max at swimming lessons. With the help of a great teacher, Alex, and his therapy, he became more comfortable and confident in the water.

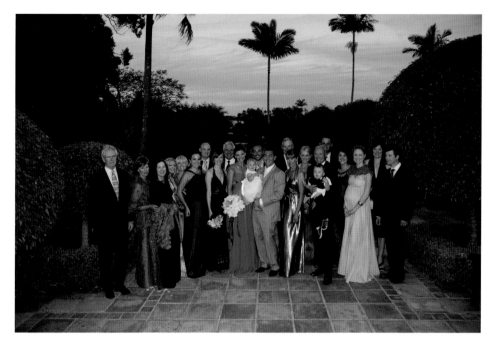

My family at our wedding. The event – like most of our life – was not without drama, but it meant so much for me and Mat to have everyone there supporting us, despite their own grievances.

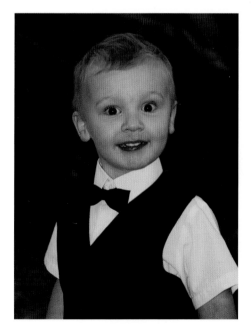

Max looked adorable in this outfit for our wedding. This was one of the few photos in which he actually looked like he was cooperating.

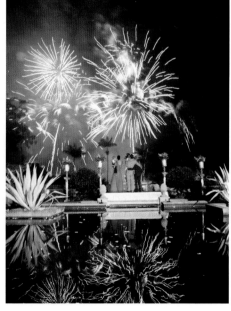

Our marriage was not just about bringing two people together, it was uniting a family. All the kids were very much involved in the wedding.

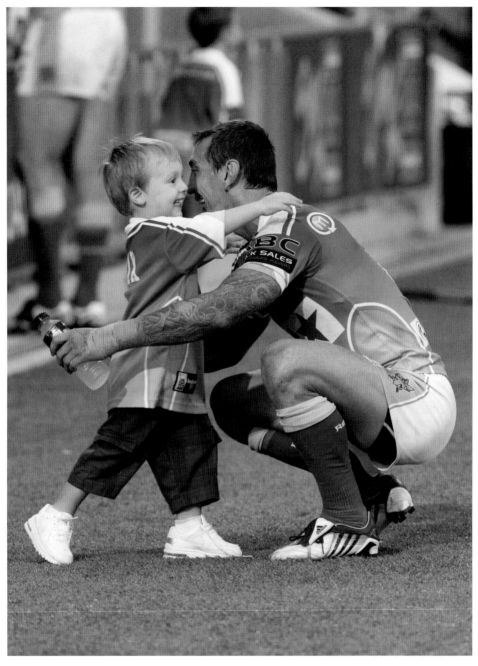

Max running out to give Mat a hug after a Titans' home game. Mat loved having the kids run on after a game, especially if the team had won!

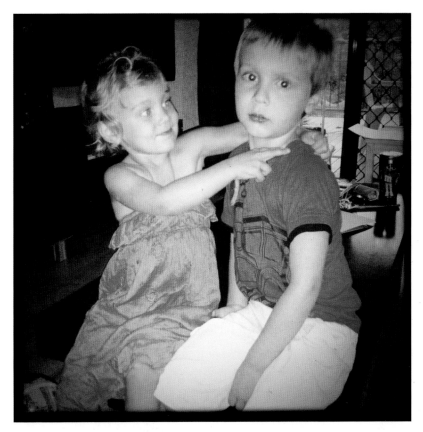

Phoenix was born 15 months after Max and has never treated him differently. He doesn't like having his photo taken and she always forces him out of his comfort zone.

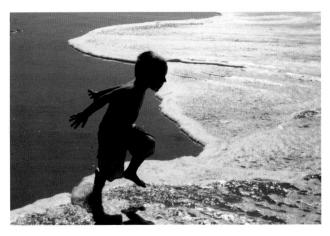

Max at the beach at the end of our street at Mermaid. He was more than a bit apprehensive about moving, but eventually came to really love our place and the ocean.

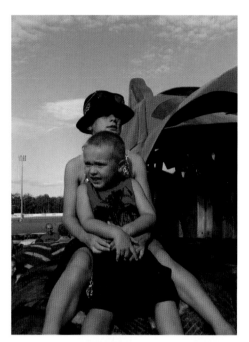

Max and Skyla at the monster trucks at Parklands on the Gold Coast. He still doesn't like having his photo taken, but we have learnt to make him comfortable and surround him with familiar objects.

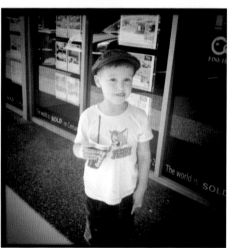

Max down at our local shops in 2010 at Mermaid Beach. He dressed himself that day and I was so proud of him — a major achievement! He loves Tom and Jerry and slurpees.

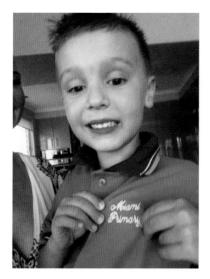

Max's first day of school; I never dared to picture this day. After almost three years of therapy, he was able to attend a local state school. I hear he is very popular with the ladies!

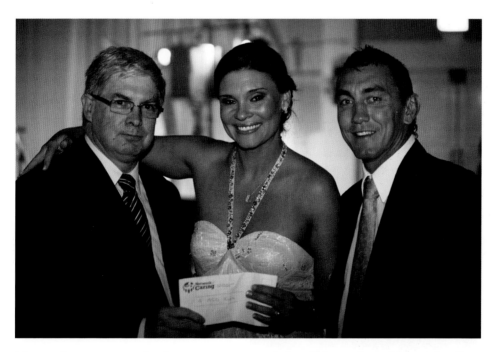

Mat and me at our gala charity evening with Ian Abbott, from Network of Caring. Network of Caring is a great supporter of our charity, 4ASDkids.

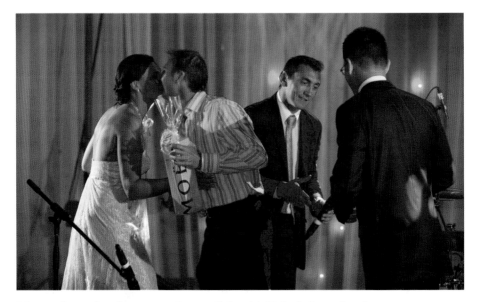

Mat and me thanking members of the 4ASDkids board, who give up their time and resources to help others. Mat left for the hospital shortly after this moment to be treated for carbon monoxide poisoning!

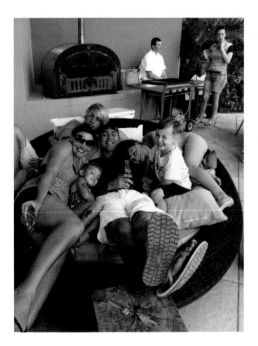

The whole family at a BBQ. It's moments like these when we are all together that Mat and I absolutely cherish. Myself, Phoenix, Jack, Mat, Skyla and Max.

16

No single story would they find
Of an unbroken happy mind,
A finish worthy of the start.

— W.B. Yeats, 'Why Should Not Old Men Be Mad?'

Max only saw the people he wanted to see. He could see Mat and me, but if visitors came, he would stare straight through them. Even if they walked right up to him and said, 'Hi, Max, how are you doing?' there would be absolutely no reaction — it was as if it simply hadn't happened. I know many kids seem to have selective hearing — blocking out anything that doesn't involve words like 'chocolate' and 'park' — but with Max, it was as though he had selective sight.

I used to think I was going mad most of the time with Max. I really had no idea just how difficult he was relative to other children, though: I simply thought this was normal behaviour for a little boy, until one day everything clicked into place in my mind.

Dad and Jo were visiting for the week and we had decided to go to the surf club at Burleigh Heads for lunch. It was a busy Saturday afternoon and there were people everywhere: families carrying foldout chairs, towels and umbrellas down to the beach, kids throwing sand at each other and having a ball. It truly was a beautiful summer Gold Coast day, the perfect day to have lunch at the beach.

As soon as we walked into the club Max seemed very uneasy. He tried to turn straight around and go back to the car, but I softly encouraged him inside. 'C'mon, mate, it's OK,' I said in the calmest voice possible.

The club was very busy. There were kids running around and families everywhere eating big hamburgers and hot chips. Max zeroed in on a support railing running beside the wheelchair access ramp leading down into the restaurant. He marched straight up to it, held on as tight as he could and refused to let go.

Rather than cause a scene in front of all of these people I let him be and we ordered some food. 'Please just behave enough so I can have a nice meal with Dad and Jo,' I thought, looking over at this bizarre child.

In contrast, Phoenix was making herself very comfortable indeed. She had plopped herself down on the ground with some other kids she had immediately made friends with, and was drawing with some crayons supplied by the staff to keep kids busy while their parents ate. Every now and then she would look over at Max attached to the railing with a quizzical look on her face, as if to say, 'How can you think that pole is more fun than these kids and these crayons?'

Max was clearly distressed and not enjoying being there at all. Our food arrived and I tried to coax him over to the table with some hot chips and soft drink. It worked. He very reluctantly came over, staring around him wide-eyed as though he was a lamb being led to slaughter.

It was then I realised he had soiled his nappy. Excusing myself, I picked him up to take him through the poker machine room and into the bathroom. 'I wonder if there's a change table in the toilet?' I speculated out loud. More often in these places there wasn't and mums are forced to change their babies on the ground.

Max was reasonably quiet until the lights and sounds of the poker machines triggered something within him akin to absolute terror. He erupted into high-pitched screams as though I had taken a butcher's knife to him and was murdering him. I later found out that his condition is very sensory. Sounds, lights and smells can overwhelm him: whereas a typically developed kid can block out a fair amount of sensory stimulation, his senses are acutely enhanced. Everyone in the whole place turned around and frowned at this brat of a child who wouldn't do as he was told and was causing a horrific scene. I eventually pushed him into the disabled toilet and attempted to change him on the floor, as there was no change table. Amidst the kicking, struggling and screaming that followed, the look on his face was one of pure hate. He seriously wanted to harm me and was doing his absolute darndest to do so.

Why is my son, whom I love so much, lashing out and kicking me in the face? What an excruciating feeling — to have your two-year-old look at you as though he wanted to kill you. I felt a sense of the most profound rejection mixed with utter embarrassment, as I could hear that people had suddenly grown quiet outside the door, obviously wondering why this child was carrying on so.

When I came out Dad and Jo had already paid the bill and were organising Phoenix so that we could leave. Every eye in the club was on us as people 'tsked' under their breath. I felt like ripping their judgmental eyes out of their skulls and feeding them to them. 'Would you like fries with that?' I thought to myself as I mentally ripped their eyeballs out of their sockets.

Outside, Dad and Jo thought it might calm Maxi down to go for a run along the beach, so we began walking toward the bustling shore. Max's tantrum shifted into overdrive. It was as if the sound of the ocean and all of the people were upsetting him even more. He took off, running towards the busy street. I ran after him.

'What's wrong, mate?' I asked, grabbing hold of his little arm. He began screaming and wailing in terror as I tried to coax him back towards the water.

I felt helpless. As a mother, you pride yourself on knowing what upsets your children and how to fix it. I had absolutely no idea what was going on in his head.

He ran again towards the road and the cars. A tiny but terrible part of me was hoping he would just be run over and that would be it. I was shocked at myself for thinking such a thing; at one and the same time I felt completely helpless and at the end of my tether. I can empathise with someone like Daniela Dawes in moments like these, when the stress overrides your rationality. Her stress drove her to attempted suicide after she had taken her own autistic son's life.

We finally reached him where he stood wailing in the car park. After a screaming fit like you have never seen, with cheek ripping, eye gouging and spitting, we decided it best to go home before any other people walking past felt the need to stop and stare in horror, and before I felt the need to smash their judgmental heads in with my bare fists.

'He's just too difficult, Chloe!' Jo said to me and I nodded tearfully.

I sobbed in the car the whole way home, with Max and Phoenix looking on from the back seat. My son is not normal, I have failed as a mother — what do I do? God, please just let us know what is wrong!

Many times with Max I felt like giving up, but I knew there had to be a solution. Anyone who knows me knows that I don't quit on anything. There has to be an answer somewhere for everything.

I had started taking Max to a speech therapist in the hope that this may somehow help his speech develop. Before he gave me any answers on Max's condition, the paediatrician recommended it and sent us to a lady by the name of Margaret. She operated her business out of a room that appeared to be attached to the back of her house. The room was tiny and contained only a little table and chairs for the kids to sit at and her desk. In the hallway to the room were boxes of toys and files and a photocopying machine.

Maxi went to see her once a week. This was not something he ever enjoyed; however, she was instrumental in getting a written diagnosis that would enable us to access the right therapies to help Max get ahead.

I would pull off the busy road into Margaret's driveway; Max would begin wriggling with anxiety in his baby seat as soon as he recognised where he was. His grumbling noises started off as little grunts but the closer we got to the door at the side of the building the louder and more pronounced they would become. Often we would have to wait for Margaret to finish with someone else before we could go in, another thing that incensed Max. He wanted to open the door and go straight into where he knew the toys were as soon as he got there, otherwise he would have a major tantrum. This particular day we had arrived on time but Margaret was running a little late finishing off with a young girl and her parents before us. Hearing the young girl and Margaret running through their exercises, I tried to tiptoe up the side path with Max. Max's grunting escalated to fever pitch: he seemed to be competing with the noises we could hear through the door.

'Max — be quiet please, mate,' I requested in my calmest voice. He continued to grunt out his aggravation. I pushed him down onto a chair outside the door and, sitting next to him, tried to restrain him by putting my hand on his leg. He grabbed hold of my arm and dug his nails in as hard as he could. I bit my lip and tried not to scream. He was too strong for me: pushing my arm off, he dashed across to the other door and flung it open with all his might. Inside the therapy room sat a shocked-looking little girl. Her parents' faces were crimson with rage at the interruption. Margaret was trying to stay composed but I could tell she was annoyed with Max bursting in on her lesson.

'Max, I'm sorry but you will have to wait your turn,' she said.

'I'm sorry,' I said and biting my tongue with rage, took Max by the bicep and pulled him outside, closing the door behind us.

I was enraged with his behaviour but I was also furious with the lack of compassion or understanding shown by any of the adults. They had looked at me with disdain, as though I was not in control of my own child.

When Max finished his lesson with Margaret that day, it was the last one he would ever have there.

Taking Max for a blood test is without doubt the worst thing I have ever had to do as a mother. I had taken the kids for their shots in the past and that was difficult enough, but for a blood test the needle has to stay in the child's arm for much longer than the quick jab of a shot.

I knew I would need Mat's help for this one, as my little boy seemed to have superhuman strength. In the past I had had to hold Max down so the doctor could give him his immunisations. It was never easy, so I scheduled a time when Mat was available to help. From what I understood they needed to take quite a lot of blood and some urine too, as they were testing for many different things.

We arrived at the pathology practice in Southport mid-morning. 'Thank God, the waiting room is empty,' I thought to myself. 'No judgmental stares to contend with!'

I remembered vaguely a time when I was proud to take my little baby boy out in public, when people would coo-chi-coo him and tell me, 'What an adorable baby.' He used to seek out people, women mostly, and openly flirt with them, but not any more. Every public social situation with him I dreaded now as he was so unpredictable, and I knew that if Max got into one of his moods there was no way I was going to be able to bring him out of it. I often travelled with a supply of chips, lollies and cookies in a bag, in the hope that I may be able to use them to subdue him. Sometimes it worked, but not always.

A lady came out from one of the rooms and called Maxi's name. Mat and I each took one of his hands and walked into the sterile little room. As soon as we shut the door Max began getting agitated: he knew something was going on he didn't like and he began working himself up. The nurse asked us to put him on the bed so she could begin. Getting him up on that bed was like trying to push a boulder up a cliff. He was not having any of it.

'This is going to have to be quick!' Mat said through his teeth in a pained voice as he lifted a struggling Max up onto the bed and lay on top of him to hold him down. Max was kicking and screaming feverishly by now. I looked around at the happy pictures of cats and dogs on the wall, put there to ease the little minds of children. Maxi's mind was far from eased and no puppy dog was going to help, that was for sure.

'I'll try my best,' said the nurse as she fumbled for the needle. She took a painstakingly long time to get organised.

Max began writhing in fear, his eyes wide with terror.

'I need his arm held still,' the nurse squealed in an agitated voice, obviously unprepared for this vicious onslaught. Max was unnaturally strong when he went into one of his rages, so Mat had to thrust all of his eighty-five kilograms upon him in an effort to keep him still. Despite this, Max could still move, and he flailed his arms wildly. I could see the nurse trying to find a vein and missing several times. I felt sick watching my baby's arm becoming a pincushion for a nurse who clearly had little experience with children when it came to taking blood, let alone a child on the spectrum.

Eventually she managed to extract one vial-full before Max momentarily wriggled free and smacked her in the arm. She reeled with shock, clutching the blood-filled vial.

'You're going to have to bring him back another time,' she said, wiping a bead of sweat from her brow and clearly unnerved. She put a sticky label on the vial, scribbled on it and placed it ever so carefully in a sealed plastic bag to be sent off to the laboratory.

'He is extremely distressed and I just don't think I can do any more today, but I do need to take more blood,' she explained apologetically.

'Bring him back?' I mouthed to Mat when the nurse's back was turned. Mat shook his head, clearly deflated. His shoulders hunched as he picked Max up and delicately stroked his tear-stained cheek. I think Mat was shocked by what had happened in this little room. He very rarely saw the tensions that I dealt with each day. Even going to the grocery store could be a major battle with Max, but when Mat came home at the end of a day's training, all he could see was his adorable if slightly high-maintenance little boy. So this whole experience had been decidedly traumatic for him. What father wants to have to restrain his son physically in order to inflict pain on him? I could see the hurt play across his face. He flashed his eyes at me sadly and then slowly carried Max out the door, past the happy puppy and the happy kitty cat, to our car outside. The blood test results ended up proving Max had no allergies whatsoever to gluten and casein. so the whole experience had been superfluous and would always just serve as a horrible memory.

* * *

When I finally got that dreaded written diagnosis, I was told by the paediatrician to contact an autism advisor. These are people employed by the government in order to best advise you on funding and therapies available for your special needs child. It was actually a good thing that we had a written diagnosis, despite the crushing emotions that came with it. Having that piece of paper meant that my little boy would have access to all the therapies he needed to move forward. He would also have access to what the government called 'the autism care package'. This meant that some of the funding for Max's therapies would be taken care of.

We arranged to meet our autism advisor at a facility in Arundel, at the other end of the Gold Coast from our new home in Mermaid Beach, where we had moved to be closer to the beach. The facility was called 'Little Souls Taking Big Steps'.

We discovered later that Little Souls is a childcare facility that caters for typically developed children as well as those with an autism spectrum disorder. By this stage, I had read enough to know that 'typically developed' was the politically correct terminology. 'Normal' meant that the autistic kids must then be considered 'not normal', and I wasn't having that.

The building was right on the corner of a busy road. It had a big sign that read 'Little Souls Taking Big Steps' showing two children made out of the soles of feet. Two little footprints with faces. 'A double entendre — very cute,' I thought to myself, not yet ready to be too impressed by anything.

Mat and I pulled into the car park, which was almost full of cars. The advisor had asked that Max come with us, so we had both the two little ones. We couldn't bring one and not the other, so Phoenix tagged along too. At the entrance we were buzzed in through a security door. At the front desk we were greeted by a smiling young woman, who motioned for us to sign in while she let our autism advisor know we were here. The counter was littered with flyers for charity events, government brochures and notices for parents.

Within minutes we were greeted by another smiling young woman, who introduced herself.

'Hello, I'm Ren and this is my assistant.' We followed her in to one of the day-care rooms. I could hear screams of delight coming from the other end of the hallway. There were a lot of kids enjoying themselves down there, I thought.

Looking around the empty day-care room, I saw there was a large glass sliding door with an awesome outdoor play area beyond it. Hanging from a piece of string across the ceiling were finger paintings, hundreds of multicoloured fingerprints from many different little hands. One corner of the room was lined with shelves full of children's books and arranged with colourful beanbags. Another had pigeonholes with hats in them and different names on each, obviously for the children to wear outside. There were toys galore stacked up in another corner and a bathroom with a baby change table and three little toilets for little people.

Max's and Phoenix's eyes grew big, taking in their new

surroundings and all of the new toys. Ren opened the glass sliding door for them to go outside; needing no encouragement whatsoever, they almost bowled her over to get out there. Laughing and giggling, Max and Phoenix were loving this. I immediately felt sure that this was a great place for kids.

Then Danielle from Autism Queensland, our autism advisor, came in to greet us. 'Please take a seat.' She gestured to two school chairs. Mat and I sat down and looked at her expectantly. I had brought a folder of every document pertaining to Max.

'Do you have the diagnosis?' Danielle asked, looking at my folder.

'Yes,' I replied, nervously fumbling through all of the different sheets in my folder until I found the right one. Mat seemed impressed by my folder. I was organised, if nothing else.

Handing that once-dreaded piece of paper over to her, I glanced out the window. There was Max trying to pedal a three-wheeler bike. After a few failed attempts of pedalling he gave up and just began running while sitting on it to make it move. His little face had the biggest smile on it I had seen in a long time. There was my little boy. For a split second I saw him again. He was blissfully unaware that inside this little room we were planning how we could turn his life around for the better. My heart began to brim with newfound hope.

Over the next hour Danielle talked us through some different options for Max that fell under the autism care package supplied by the government.

'You could do home care,' she said, looking over the top of her glasses at us as her assistant took notes quietly in the corner. Mat and I looked at each other, puzzled as to what that might mean.

'Someone would come to your house to give Max therapy and they would basically train you so you could eventually carry out your own therapy. Kind of like home-schooling,' Danielle explained.

That sounded very overwhelming to me. I was struggling enough as it was with the day-to-day grind of caring for Max, let alone trying to give him therapy myself. There were days when I wouldn't leave the house because it was all too hard. It was a constant mental and emotional drain trying to figure out Max — what he wanted, why he was attacking me, why he seemed to want to kill me. Mat was training six days a week, so it would all come down to me. Not to mention that Phoenix would be at home too and the other two, Jack and Skyla, were coming up to stay in the school holidays.

I was exhausted at the thought. Mat was very supportive but he was also a professional athlete who was required to work six days out of seven. I did not feel confident with that responsibility on my own.

'What are our other options?' I enquired, feeling that if my eyes closed right now I would have real trouble opening them again. I was feeling more and more lethargic every day without a clear path for my Maxi. One thing I knew from everything I had read was that we needed to begin Maxi's therapy fast in order for him to have any semblance of a regular life later on. Early intervention was crucial for these kids to be broken out of their quirky routines. The earlier the better. Every day Max was not getting therapy I reckon I grew another grey hair thinking about it.

'There are several facilities like the one we're in today that cater to autistic children's specific needs in terms of early intervention,' she replied, sensing the reaction to the first option was a definite no.

'Early intervention, particularly at Little Souls, has a seventy per cent success rate of children going on to normal schools without requiring much assistance,' Danielle said, looking out the window at Phoenix trying to encourage Max to play with her.

Mat and I looked at each other, nodding in silent agreement. 'So … he can come here?' asked Mat.

'Yes, this is a facility we endorse. He would be here five days a week doing four hours of what we call ABA therapy a day.'

My prayers had been answered. He could come here. He would get the help he needed and I would have some much-needed respite.

'When can he start?' I asked, rejoicing that we may have found the answer.

'Well, I can check with Robyn — she's the founder of Little Souls.' Danielle looked toward her assistant, who stood and went out to find Robyn.

The advisor didn't need to say it but we could tell she thought this was the best place for Max. 'It will be rather expensive, because he'll have one-on-one therapy,' she said, scribbling notes in her notepad.

'Whatever it takes,' replied Mat.

'God I love him!' I thought to myself.

The assistant returned with Robyn Hawkins, the founder of Little Souls, someone from whom we were to draw great inspiration in the future. She assured us that Max could be put on the list and he could probably start in a few months.

Finding Little Souls was such a relief to me. Max's care had been weighing heavily on my shoulders, and I was far from confident I was the right person to manage his therapy. This place had such a gorgeous vibe, with children playing happily and staff who seemed to really care and were used to dealing with ASD kids day in, day out. I felt a renewed sense of energy and of confidence that Little Souls would be the right place to bring Max.

This was the real beginning of our fight for our son's identity. I knew it was in there somewhere — I'd seen it in the early days. Now we were going into battle to drag Max out of that distant world into which he had withdrawn.

17

One that is ever kind said yesterday:
'Your well-belovéd's hair has threads of grey,
And little shadows come about her eyes;
Time can but make it easier to be wise
Though now it seems impossible, and so
All that you need is patience.'

— W.B. Yeats, 'The Folly of Being Comforted'

For so long it seemed as if Max was just a vessel with nothing going on inside. But I knew there was something more in there somewhere, we just needed to draw it out.

Once we started seeking out more information to help Max, it seemed everywhere we turned someone had an opinion to offer. The internet is overflowing with advice from so many different sources, as I had found out in the early days. There is so much information out there about autism spectrum disorders it's hard to know what's relevant to your child and what's not. There was also, it appeared, a never-ending stream of knowledge to be had from family members, friends and acquaintances. Everyone was an expert on what we should be doing. They were all extremely well meaning, of course, but I eventually decided that I simply couldn't keep running around trying to carry out everyone's suggestions.

The team doctor for the Titans, Dr Paul Ohmsen, was very well-respected by the players and in the Gold Coast community. Mat had gotten to know him quite well over his time with the Titans due to the countless injuries he had suffered from season to season. Paul mentioned to Mat one day that his wife Jay was a special educator and very familiar with cases like Max's. He said that she had offered to have a chat with us if we needed it. With our last paediatrician visit still rankling in my mind, I decided to call Jay and ask her advice.

Jay turned out to be an absolute breath of fresh air. She spoke to me with a sincere sense of understanding of what I was going through. There was no condescending tone in her voice but a great deal of empathy and patience as I described my current predicament. Jay suggested that Max attend an SEDU (Special Education Department Unit) class once a week at Burleigh Heads State School, ten minutes drive from our home. This way he would immediately be in some sort of program while we decided what program he was best suited for, longer term. These programs are state funded so they're free for special needs kids to attend with their parents. It allows them to socialise with other kids and prepares them for a classroom environment. Initially, kids go along with mum or dad once a week and then as they become more comfortable they can attend without their parents a few times a week. Jay was in charge of the SEDU unit at Burleigh Heads, so she knew what a difference the classes can make for autistic children — and for the parents too.

It was fantastic for me to get to speak to other mothers in a similar situation. The kids attending had issues ranging from Down's syndrome to autism and cerebral palsy, and they were all preschool age. The mothers I met there were inspirational. I was heartbroken to see babies with crippling ailments in some cases but at the same time incredibly encouraged by the strength these women possessed. They were doing the best they could for their children and doing it really tough, but in their eyes you could see a glimmer of hope and a fire of expectancy for the future. It was contagious, I loved it.

Our extended family had eventually settled in to the knowledge that Max was going to need a little extra help. We had already overcome so much as a family and individually, it was now time to work together to overcome this next hurdle. They decided to take it in turns coming up to support me. Each of them had now gone through all of the emotional stages that I had also gone through at the start, they had found out more about autism and what it really meant, and now they had made it through to the proactive stage. I was grateful and more than ready to move on from the past in order to ensure Max's future.

My brother Brodie came up and spent a week with us when he was in between jobs. He really was amazing: he vacuumed, took the kids to the beach when I needed a break, and offered me a shoulder to cry on in between appointments.

One Monday I took Brodie along to Maxi's SEDU class. I don't think he had any idea of what to expect. Phoenix would always come with me, since she was not in childcare and I had no family on the Gold Coast to look after her. She loved it, though, and the staff were very accepting of her being there. This particular morning we arrived at the SEDU, a cream-coloured building at the back of Burleigh Heads State School, before all the other kids. Phoenix and Max ran for all of their favourite toys as soon as we entered. Brodie was scanning the room, taking in the abundance of activities for the kids to do. I wondered how he would respond to the other kids when they arrived. If you're not used to it, seeing one or two special needs kids is not as shocking as seeing a whole bunch of them together in the one room. The first time I came to the SEDU I was overwhelmed with seeing so many disabilities. Little children should not have to be in this situation, I remember thinking.

Soon enough the other parents began filtering in with their children. Brodie, who had been engrossed in a game with Phoenix, looked up to greet them with a smile but his face noticeably fell. Autistic kids look like every other kid, they just act different, but it's immediately evident when a kid has cerebral palsy or Down's syndrome. There was one child in particular, a little boy aged around one year, who was very clearly impeded. His eyes were rolled back in his head and saliva collected on his bib as his mouth hung limply open. When he was wheeled in, Brodie looked close to tears. Another little girl with metal braces on her legs came limping in, clearly excited to see the other kids despite her serious impairment. Max played on, oblivious to the children around him. He was totally in his own world. Phoenix, on the other hand, was keen to try to interact with the other kids, but to no avail in most cases. Autistic kids don't tend to relate with others — they prefer to play on their own — and the cerebral palsy kids were not very active.

'Twinkle, Twinkle, Little Star' began vibrating through an extremely old stereo system. That meant it was group time and all of the kids were expected to sit on the carpet. Phoenix would run and sit down straight away, excited to see what was happening next. She was so keen that she would often begin an activity before the teacher started it. I sometimes worried that her presence might be a constant reminder to the other parents of just how far behind their kids were — she was so much more advanced developmentally.

Max didn't like group time at all. He would kick and scream and have a massive tantrum to avoid sitting on the carpet. Most of the autistic kids reacted to group time in this way. They would either have tantrums or they would just get up, block their ears and walk away on tiptoes to play on their own. ('Toe walking' is one of the common behaviours associated with autism, along with hand flapping and finger gazing.)

The mothers and children all gathered in a semicircle, sitting on whatever seats we could find. Max sat for a few seconds, but only because of me forcing him, and then leapt up with a high-pitched scream and ran to the other side of the room. I walked over to get him and he punched and kicked me.

'Just leave him for now, Chloe,' Jay said to me softly. 'He'll get used to it eventually.' I was agitated that Max couldn't carry out a simple task like sitting and listening. This was a common experience in my role as 'Max's mother'.

When the session was over, we headed out to the car. Phoenix did not want to leave but Max was well and truly ready to go.

'Goodbye, everyone.' I tried to coax Max into waving to the other kids. He simply walked straight out to the car park and did not look back. Phoenix turned and waved sweetly to those children still remaining.

As we drove home, Brodie sat quietly for some time. He eventually turned to me, his eyes glistening.

'Max doesn't belong there.' I saw a single tear slide along the rim of his eye.

'He needs to be somewhere, Brods,' I said, half agreeing but also half afraid that I may never find anywhere that was right for him. I hoped that Little Souls would be that right place I was searching for. The future was so scary and so unknown, but I did feel better to have someone like Jay to confide in. I would often stay back after the class to talk with her about some behaviour of Max's that I didn't know how to handle, and over time she came to be an important part of my support network.

After a few months on the waiting list, Max finally started at Little Souls Taking Big Steps. For us, it really wasn't that difficult getting him in there as we were one of a few families that had the money. We could afford it. A lot of other families were on the waiting list for much longer — for them it was the 'waiting-till-we-can-afford-it' list. Including the childcare element, the annual fees amounted to between $30,000 and $40,000, which is more than the fees for even the most elite private schools. The Australian government gives you an allowance (the Helping Children with Autism support payment) once your child is diagnosed, which is approximately $12,000 over two years. Clearly, that was not even going to touch the sides of my wallet, let alone cover the entire costs of Maxi's childcare and therapy. Thankfully we were blessed with a high income between us. Many others were not so lucky. For most families, having a child on the spectrum means one parent must become a full-time carer; $6,000 a year doesn't come close to replacing that loss of income, even before the additional therapy costs.

Five days a week, Monday to Friday, I would drop Max off at Little Souls at eight in the morning. He absolutely hated me leaving him at first. It was such a new environment for him and he really did not like unfamiliar people or environments.

Every morning we would pull into the car park and Max would realise where we were straight away. 'Noooooooo!' He would begin to writhe and moan in his car seat.

I would undo his straps and he would scramble across to the other side of the car. I would run around the back of the car only to find he had crossed over again. This would go on and on, until finally I would just lean across and grab him by his t-shirt. I would pretty much have to drag him into the building and try to wrestle open the door while carrying Max and his school bag as well. Once signed in and inside the kindy room, he would immediately go and find a table and hide under it. The therapists told me that this would be where he would remain for several hours, not moving a muscle, as though he were in a self-induced coma.

The school had one big kindy room where typically developed kids and autistic kids mingled together. They all practised what they call 'functional play' with each other and ate their lunch and morning tea together. I thought this was fantastic: I wanted Max to have some typically developed role models to imitate.

The autistic children in the centre also had their own individual rooms to which they would be taken for one-on-one therapy with their therapists. Max's therapist would practically have to remove him surgically from under his table in order to coerce him up to the therapy room. Two therapists were assigned to each child and they would work with the child separately, one for two hours in the morning and one for two hours in the afternoon.

The therapists at Little Souls practised applied behavioural analysis (ABA) therapy, which was much criticised in the autistic community — wrongly, I believe. Some professionals did not agree with the way ABA therapy relied on positive reinforcement, rewarding progress with treats such as cookies, lollies and chips. I say whatever works, and work it did. After the first few weeks my little boy was coming along in leaps and bounds. I do know that this sort of therapy is not necessarily beneficial for every child on the spectrum but it worked absolute miracles for our son.

One of Max's therapists was Carla, who was the sweetest girl. He really warmed to her straight away. I liked her because she was so warm and patient with him. His other therapist was Maria, who was Greek. I remember one day I was playing with Max and we had just put together a train track.

'All finished,' I said.

He looked me in the eye and replied, 'Vary good!' in a distinct Greek accent. The next day I took him into the kindy room, where he was greeted by Maria and taken to the bathroom. Upon finishing I heard Maria say, 'Vary good,' in exactly the same tone. I chuckled to myself and wondered if my little boy would one day develop his own tone and spontaneous sense of humour.

In those first days at Little Souls, some mornings were a nightmare for Max; he would have the most incredible tantrums and screaming fits. I would find myself greeting other mums on the way out with tears on my cheeks, scratches on my face and the pain of helplessness in my eyes. I would smile and greet them and they would nod back with a knowing flicker of understanding. Those telltale gestures helped us comfort each other without even having to say a word. Words were not necessary among these women, and for that I was so grateful. I was sick of words: they reminded me of their absence in my son.

Other days Max would be great and it would be another mum wrestling with her child in the car park. Often a mum could be found in the kindy room pinning down their child with the help of a therapist while tears streamed down their cheeks and the child writhed in anger and confusion. It was all part of the process. Patience was something all of us mums with ASD kids had to learn. Progress does come eventually, but a plateau in development can follow closely behind, so the process can be long, drawn-out and painful. I believe it was Thoreau who once said success is not a destination but its journey. The bigger the struggle in that journey then the bigger the prize, I reminded myself over and over again through those early days as we fought to draw Max out of his bubble.

18

Never had I more
Excited, passionate, fantastical
Imagination, nor an ear and eye
That more expected the impossible …

— W.B. Yeats, 'The Tower'

We had been trying to keep Max's condition a secret from the media for some time. We weren't yet ready to speak out loud about what was happening because we had to get our heads around what we needed to put in place for the little man. There was so much overwhelming and often conflicting information out there that we wanted to make sure we had it together as a couple first. According to an article in the *Journal of Family Psychology*, studies find that parents of children with autism are more likely to get divorced than parents of children with no developmental disabilities. We wanted to be confident within ourselves and able to stand strong as a unit before we faced the onslaught of the outside world.

We didn't talk directly about the risk that this might tear our family apart, but it was always unspoken between us that it would be better to face it together than separately. Looking back, I can see that Mat was more supportive to me than I gave him credit for at the time. I remember him coming with me to a series of workshops for families dealing with ASD: at the very first one, he was ready to walk out halfway through. Mat has always been about maintaining a positive attitude in every aspect of his life, and many parents there were very angry about how little the government was doing for them and felt very victimised. For Mat, that was a completely alien way of seeing things and I suspect it was very confronting for him. To his credit, he stayed put through the whole session — and went back the next week.

One thing we learnt through the passing of Mat's father Steve was that even the most well-meant gestures from strangers can be difficult to cope with. When people know who you are and what you are going through personally, everyone has an opinion or unintentionally reminds you of what you don't necessarily want to be reminded about. We needed to strengthen up mentally before all of that began again. It had been only a few years since Steve had passed and now we were facing another crisis. It's one thing dealing with the reality of having an autistic child in the privacy of your own home and your own life, and yet another dealing with it in the public eye.

One day we got a call from Danny Weidler, a friend who knew our situation. He was also a sports journalist for Channel Nine. He asked if we would do a story for the Channel Nine news about little Max and what we were going through. I really didn't want to do a story just for the sake of a story, so we said no. But some time later, after reading a lot of material on ASD and meeting a lot of mums and families through Little Souls, I decided we had an opportunity to turn a negative situation into a positive.

Talking to other mothers of children with autism, what I kept hearing was that one-on-one therapy was incredibly expensive. Many of the parents I had met through the SEDU would never have the chance to bring their children to a facility like Little Souls because it was too costly. One couple I met at Little Souls were Di and Rob, whose son James had autism. Both of them worked, and with his job Rob would often have to go away for months at a time. It was tough for them, yet at the same time they were incredibly active in fundraising for the centre: Rob did a sponsored motorbike ride, they organised barbecues to raise money, they got the Titans involved in fundraising events. If Di and Rob could do all of that, what could we offer?

Perhaps we could use our celebrity as currency, I thought. Bono from U2 once said something along those lines in an interview — not that we were ever as famous as Bono, but people knew who we were, particularly here on the Gold Coast. We could do something on our own scale.

Max had been progressing incredibly well at Little Souls, so at last we could see light at the end of the tunnel. I had done enough reading by now to understand the importance of early intervention for these kids; where early intervention programs are accessible, the statistics of those going on to a life of independence are overwhelming. It broke our hearts that not every family could have access to these programs because of money, or a lack thereof.

Now that we were confident with where Max was and we felt stronger within ourselves, Mat and I began talking about the possibility of helping other families with a greater need who were less well-off financially than we were. When the oxygen masks drop down in an aeroplane, you're encouraged to put yours on before helping someone less able. That always seemed to me quite a selfish thing to do, until I worked out that it actually made a lot of sense. You can't help anyone else until you have helped yourself. Mat and I had our 'oxygen masks' on so now we could lend other people a hand. The idea excited us and it even brought us closer together; we felt we now had a joint purpose binding us. There was a reason God blessed us with a little boy who was different, and we now knew what that reason was. It was time to act on that.

We came up with the idea of raising funds to help kids access early intervention programs all across Australia. At the same time we wanted to educate people about ASD and what it means for children. Ignorance is the enemy of most of these kids' lives: we wanted to let people know that when they see a child acting in a particular way, there may be a very good reason for it.

So we decided to set up a sort of trust through which we could use our 'celebrity status' — I hate that term, but the reality was that we could use our profiles to raise funds to help other families who were really struggling. In other words, using our powers for good instead of evil. Aha!

We had figured out that we wanted to help other families dealing with ASD; the next step was working out how to do it. I knew we would need some help with that one, and I thought of the Classic Events Company who had organised the mega-event that was our wedding. I knew they had ties to George Gregan's foundation that helps sick children — Mat and George had played for the Wallabies together and we had supported several of their events in the past. I was sure the Classic Events team could help us too, so I called them to set up a meeting.

When we arrived at the café where we had arranged to meet, Andy Payne from Classic Events came out to greet us. He is a tall man, softly spoken, with kind eyes. Mat and I got along really well with him.

'Hey, guys,' he said, shaking Mat's hand and kissing my cheek while ushering us in through the café. Phil Harte, the owner of Classic Events, was sitting at a table at the back.

Phil wasn't a very well-liked man. Medium height with a Tom Selleck-style moustache, he had a reputation for being incredibly blunt and arrogant. He tended to rub people up the wrong way if they didn't know him well; he did, however, get things done and that was exactly what we needed.

'OK, what can we do for you?' he asked, tapping his watch as though to remind us that time was money.

Mat and I described the vision we had to help other families with ASD kids. We talked about setting up a board and a website and organising some events. Tears welled in our eyes as we shared our dream; these guys assured us it would all become a reality.

The name of our charity, 4 ASD Kids, was my little brainwave. It popped into my head one day and it just stuck.

We decided that one of the first-ever 4 ASD Kids events would be 'The Classic Week' at the Hyatt in Sanctuary Cove. The Classic Events team host this every year; it includes a massive fundraising weekend that brings together a bundle of sporting events, auctions and top-notch entertainment. It would launch 4 ASD Kids with a bang; the only thing was, the event was only six weeks away. Not a whole lot of time to organise media, sell corporate tables and get money-can't-buy auction items. We got the website up pretty quickly, but we needed media attention to make this event happen — and we needed it fast.

It was time to call Danny back.

Within days Danny flew up from Sydney to interview us about Max. As part of the story, he joined Mat and I at Little Souls to film some of Maxi's therapy. Because of Mat's six-day-a-week training commitments, he really hadn't seen much of Max in action at the centre, so I couldn't wait to show him how far our little man had come.

At eight one morning, we met Danny and his camera crew out the front of Little Souls. All of us went in and crammed into

Max's little therapy room: Mat, Danny, Max, the cameraman, Maxi's therapist Carla, and me.

Max was doing a matching exercise. 'Put cat on cat,' Carla said, handing Max a flash card with a picture of a cat on it. Max took the card and ran his eyes over the pictures on the desk. He hovered over a picture of a dog and exclaimed, 'No!' quite loudly but with a smile on his face. Then he put the cat card on top of the other cat card and said, 'Yay!'

I looked at Mat staring at our son in amazement. A single tear slid down his cheek. 'I love this man,' I thought.

The interview screened about a week later. Luckily we had the website set up by then, as we had an overwhelming response. There were so many letters from anguished families struggling with an autistic child and wanting advice, and there were letters of sincere gratitude too. Other families seemed to take solace from knowing that we were going through the same battles. Our story had given them hope that we would raise awareness as well as directly helping people who had been touched by ASD.

So many of the people who contacted us were desperate for access to early intervention programs; through Little Souls I had met a cross-section of families — like Di and Rob and their little boy James — who were also in exactly that position. These families had been hitting their heads against a brick wall before they came to the centre, but now everything had turned around and they were incredibly impressed with the results.

Every week Max astounded me with big leaps in his speech. They would have been considered pretty average leaps for a typically developed child, but for me they were huge and beyond anything I had hoped for.

Part of the parents' commitment at Little Souls is that they sit in on two hours of therapy a week and attend a fortnightly meeting to assess the child's progress. One of my first sit-ins will stay in my memory for life.

Max's therapist at this session was Maria, the very friendly Greek woman. I really liked her.

'OK, Max has been doing very well these last few weeks,' Maria said as she shuffled through her row of files next to Max's little desk.

'We're going to do some social questions now,' Maria said, finding the file she was looking for. My heart skipped a beat. These were the standard, everyday questions that you would ask a child of his age and expect a response: 'What's your name? How old are you?' and so on. The very same questions I had been answering for Max his whole life.

I had always struggled with the fact that just about every day, we would be in a situation where complete strangers would ask him, 'What's your name?' And every day I would answer for him when his silence was too much to bear: 'Max, his name is Max.' I would try to smile politely as the stranger continued on with their day, but inside a part of me would die. I felt like a failure because my son could not answer that one simple question.

I held my breath as Maria began.

'What's your name?' she asked and I bit down hard on my tongue. It had become almost a reflex for me to answer that question for him. I waited anxiously.

His little face looking straight at Maria, my child answered, 'Max.'

Our little boy had said the word, the most beautiful word in the world. His name.

My face flushed red as I tried to fight back tears of joy. I stifled a sob with my hand. I can't even begin to explain the pride. It was a feeling I would expect after watching my child win an Olympic medal, but he was simply saying his name. After everything we had been through, I never thought I would see this day.

'Good boy,' Maria said, trying not to look at me for fear of her emotions taking over too. She continued to the next question.

'Max, how old are you?' she asked.

I was already on cloud nine — how could this get any better?

'Three.' He answered so clearly I nearly fell off my chair. This was a miracle. My son, who had never really talked except for gobbledygook, was answering questions. Questions I had answered for him with the heaviest of hearts for so long.

One of the most significant and beautiful things that Max learned at Little Souls was how to respond when we told him, 'I love you.' In our family, we tell each other we love each other all the time. One of the most awesome moments in my life was the first day Max said, 'I love you', back. He had to be taught that, of course, whereas for most kids, it just comes naturally.

I left the centre exuberant that day. A feeling that had been buried deep inside me for some time was now fighting its way back up to the surface. It was hope. I had hope that our little boy could have a regular life. I couldn't wait to show Mat what he had learnt.

After a full year at Little Souls, Max had made very significant progress. He could answer a whole range of simple social questions now, such as, 'Where do you go to kindy?' and, 'What's your favourite food?' We were so excited at the prospect that our little boy would one day be able to take his place in society.

One Wednesday I was sitting in on Max's therapy with Julie, his therapist at the time, when a visiting therapist knocked on the door to the room. Sandy was a friendly woman with a Canadian accent.

'Hello, Max,' she said.

'Hello,' he replied.

'How are you today?' Sandy inquired.

'Good, thank you,' he replied. Simple, everyday stuff, but still a miracle to me.

Sandy proceeded to demonstrate a new technique Max was learning in order to deal with stress. It is very difficult for ASD kids to calm themselves down when they get worked up, so it's vital they learn stress relief techniques early so that they can control themselves as they get older. Sandy called it 'big boy relaxation'.

It involved taking him through a simple routine of deep breathing, tensing the muscles in his arms and legs and then more deep breathing. It was relatively new to Max, but he seemed to respond reasonably well to Sandy's guidance.

'How about you try now, Mum?' Sandy looked at me inquiringly.

'OK,' I replied, uncertain about how this would work out. When I came to Maxi's therapy I usually just observed and then implemented what I learnt there in Maxi's everyday home life where I could. I was not sure that he would react well to this change in routine, but I was ready to do as I was told.

'You need to use a very soft calm voice, with lots of praise,' she instructed me.

I sat down on the chair opposite Max with Julie and Sandy looking at me expectantly.

'OK, Max, deep breaths in and out,' I tried the soft voice. Max was instantly aggravated and began squirming in his seat, making loud noises of disapproval. I decided to move on to the muscle work.

'Big muscle in this arm?' I asked, pointing at his left arm. He lifted it into a flex pose but the noises became louder.

'Now relax,' I said. He began to get off his chair.

'No! No! No!' he said, rolling his eyes back in his head and grimacing at me. I hated it when he made that face. He looked like a typically developed kid most of the time until he made that face. I began to be disheartened as he lashed out, catching me in the face with his closed fist. I tried to persist but he was becoming more and more incensed with the drill.

We left it there and Sandy reassured me that with time he would respond better. Julie comforted me by telling me kids always play up more to their parents; her own daughter was no exception.

We continued on with his mixed drills. These were drills that he had done over the course of his time at Little Souls that they would revisit just to refresh his memory.

Julie put out the letters of the alphabet. I didn't remember him having done the alphabet before, so I was interested to see how he would fare with it.

'Give me A?' Julie asked Max. He looked at her blankly.

'Give me B?' she asked. After there was no response again she pulled out his 'reinforcers': Oreo cookies. More often than not when he saw that he might get a cookie, he would concentrate. He loved separating the two halves of the cookie and pulling the cream off, rolling it into a sausage and then eating it. That was his routine.

'Give me B?' she asked again, pointing at the letter this time. He gave it to her but was becoming very agitated. When she asked for C, that was it. He went into hysterics. Julie decided that the relaxation technique should be used at this point, so she began implementing what Sandy had shown her. Max, however, did not agree. When she asked him to give her deep breaths and demonstrated with her mouth, he lurched at her and smacked her in the face. We could hear the blow from his clenched fist.

Julie was very calm and persisted, but I was completely mortified. Many times I had been the victim of an attack like that from my son, but I was utterly shocked to see him treat someone else that way. She tried again.

'Deep breath, Maxi, it's alright,' she said with a loving smile on her face and the calmest of voices.

Thwack! He smacked her again, this time even harder than before. She looked up at me as I covered my mouth with both hands in shock.

'It's OK, Chloe,' she said, so calmly. 'It's good that you see him like this because in two weeks he will have come so far.

'We get paid to not react,' Julie explained gently. 'If my daughter did that to me the whole of Southport would hear about it.' She looked back at Max as he slowly began to calm down.

'Do you want to go outside and play now?' she asked him.

'No! ABCs!' he shrieked, bashing the letters with the same fist he had struck Julie with just minutes earlier.

'He wants to learn them,' Julie said. 'He's frustrated that he doesn't know the answers.'

She was right. My little boy was desperate to learn.

I could see now that this was a recurring theme in Max's life. He would get so frustrated over his lack of comprehension, which showed that he desperately wanted to improve. My son was as determined to learn as I was to see him learn.

19

That civilisation may not sink,
Its great battle lost …

— W.B. Yeats, 'Long-legged Fly'

Every time my son doesn't live up to normal expectations, a part of me dies. I've always wanted to be the best mother I could be, and even now I still sometimes blame myself for Max's failure to develop typically. I cringe every time we're at a playground or at a park and a little girl asks, 'What's wrong with that boy?' as Max wails, clutching himself and staring out into nothingness.

Every parent wants to boast about their child, wants to be proud. Sometimes I feel like Max isn't even there most of the time, let alone achieving milestones that we can be proud of. He's inside a bubble, just floating around in his own world. Every now and then he will reach out of the bubble and engage with us, but most of the time he is in a parallel universe. I find myself wondering what goes on in his head. What internal dialogues run through his mind — or does that not happen for Max? How does he talk to himself in there when he can't talk to us here in the outside world?

We could be at our neighbour's house with the kids running around having an absolute ball, but Max will refuse to get off the computer and play with any of them. Phoenix, on the other hand, is running around, playing hide-and-seek, screaming and shooting the boys with water pistols. The only sound that comes from Max is an occasional wailing noise when something goes wrong with the computer.

'I don't really know Max,' the little girl from next door once said to me. 'I've said hello to him in the front yard but he doesn't remember me or something,' she said so innocently. My heart sank.

'Max is a little bit different to other kids, sweetie.' I would come to use this sentence more times than I care to remember and every time my heart would break.

Just when I thought he was improving, he would go backwards.

It was Jack's semifinal match for the Burleigh Bears under-14s team. Just the day before, Jack had received a contract from the Gold Coast Titans and he was over the moon. They had signed him up for a two-year development deal, which meant he would be groomed to become a part of the Titans squad. Mat and I were so ridiculously proud of him. Even though I didn't give birth to Jack, I treated him as though he was my own son. I can't take the credit like his mum Michelle can, but I could still be so proud to see the amazing man he was becoming. One Rogers' career was coming to an end as another was beginning.

Jack was playing his semifinal in Beaudesert, one hour inland from the Gold Coast. When we finally got to the field, it was bedlam. There were kids everywhere and of course they all spotted Mat straight away. He was mobbed for photos and autographs. It was like this pretty much everywhere we went: he was the idol of every little boy and every man on the Gold Coast. We were very proud of him. As we walked in surrounded by people, Maxi's eyes widened. He glanced from side to side, already looking distressed.

Mat eventually finished his hero duties and caught up with us. 'I'm going to strap Jack's sternum guard on,' he said, kissing me and making his way to the sheds.

I spotted a stand selling slushies and headed over to it with the kids, figuring that if I could get something Max enjoys into his hands quickly, we could go and sit down somewhere without too much stress.

'Ice blocks, yummy!' I exclaimed, pointing at the colourful handmade slushies that were being distributed by a couple of older ladies with big smiles. Max and Phoenix pushed their way to the front of the line. I apologised profusely to everyone and pulled them back to wait our turn at the back of the line.

'What colours do you want, Maxi? Blue and purple?' I asked.

'Blue and purple,' he mimicked absent-mindedly as usual.

'What about you, Phoenix?'

'Pink and yellow,' she answered unprompted, understanding the question straight away.

I handed Phoenix hers and then Max's was ready.

'Here you go, mate,' I said cheerfully, hoping this would disperse his feelings of distress. He took the cup of coloured ice but was clearly unimpressed. I led them both away as Max began to make his wailing noises of disapproval.

'What's up, mate?' I asked in a calm voice once we found a spot to sit. He answered me with more intense wailing.

'Look Max!' I exclaimed excitedly, grabbing his slushy and using the spoon to put it into my mouth, thinking maybe he didn't know how to eat this kind of ice treat. This incensed him even more. His wailing got louder. The people around us were trying to watch a football game, but they all turned around to stare at this brat of a child.

'C'mon, mate, eat your icy,' I tried again in a calm voice and gestured to the slushy.

'Maxi, eat da icy!' Phoenix screamed at Max. He responded by kicking her in the leg and screaming louder and louder. She screamed back at him, then it was on. He was kicking and punching her and she was giving it back to him. Mat was way over the other side of the field helping Jack get ready for his game, which would start straight after the one that was being played right now. I had to sort this kid out on my own.

Think, Chloe, what was his usual routine with something like this? I thought about ice blocks I had given him before and

Slurpees, which were his favourite thing. That's why I thought he would love these. Slurpees … of course, when he has a Slurpee he eats it with a straw, not a spoon.

'Do you want a straw, Max?' I asked.

His eyes lit up. 'Straw,' he mimicked, finally finding the word he wanted. 'Yes!'

Relief flooded my entire body. He wants a straw. After twenty minutes of wailing, beating up his sister and generally annoying everyone around us, I finally worked out it was because he needed a straw.

'C'mon, let's go get a straw,' I said, motioning toward the canteen. I could see everyone around us was relieved that we were moving somewhere else.

These meltdowns happened often. Max's inability to communicate what was wrong led to so many draining episodes for me. Some weeks I had a lot of tolerance, others I thought I was on the verge of a breakdown. I would often have the most horrible thoughts about him in my head. I love my son no matter what, but when you are at the end of your tether bad thoughts creep in. Was I going insane?

We got a straw and Max was calm again — for now, anyway.

Children are incredible recorders but not great interpreters. We remember everything from our childhood: we can replay every word at will, but it's not until we have some life experience behind us that we can interpret why things happened, why certain words were used and understand the reasoning behind them.

Growing up, I went through a pretty tough time when my parents broke up. I was still emotionally scarred well into my twenties; by then I had been carrying a lot of baggage for too long and I was tired of lugging it around. But at that point I still had a massive ego and was incredibly self-centred; it wasn't until I had children of my own that I was able to grow into humility. It took becoming a mother for me to realise that it's not about me at all. I was beginning to respect who my mother was more and more with this realisation. And it's actually more rewarding when it's not about you, I find.

All of these years later, the situation is reversed and I find myself the 'evil stepmother' in a blended family. Things like that happen for a reason: I know only too well what the children in our family are going through, as I have been in their shoes. I've also been on both sides of the parent equation, which allows me to interpret my own parents' actions differently. Now I realise how difficult it is to know the best way to handle these situations. I still have more apologising to do with Mum, Dad, Ross and Jo for being so incredibly insensitive and out of control for so long — not just as a child but well into early adulthood.

Mat and I made a promise to ourselves that we would never speak badly about Mat's ex-wife in front of the kids. We may have had some heated discussions when they were not around, but these discussions were necessary so that we could be unified in decisions that would affect our whole family. We're firm believers in letting kids be kids, and not making them privy to the adult goings-on in their lives. The minute we denigrated their mum they would take it on board — and I knew that because I had used my parents' volatile situation as an excuse for my wild behaviour, many times.

Mat and his ex, Michelle, married very young and had children pretty much straight away — as did we, but Mat and I were twenty-nine when Max came along. There's a world of difference between twenty-one and twenty-nine, especially when it comes to raising children together. I know that their relationship, as volatile as it still was and can be to this day, could cause huge problems with Jack and Skyla later on. So I made it my mission to try and mend the hurt, and to give back the respect and acknowledgment Michelle deserved. That may sound completely over the top when I put it that way, but she had done a wonderful job of mothering two precious little people in my life. She was very important to them and therefore she had to be very important to us too.

One weekend, back before Phoenix was born, we were back in Cronulla. The Titans had played the Sharks that day and we had picked up Jack and Skyla so that they could stay with us at our hotel. Mat and I were lounging around our hotel room; he was watching sport on television and I was reading *Don't Sweat the Small Stuff* by Richard Carlson. When I came to a sentence that said something like, 'It is better to be kind than to be right', I had an epiphany.

'You have to go and apologise to Michelle for the way you treated her and work through all of your stuff.' It just came out of nowhere. Mat was slightly taken aback. Midway through a bowl of spaghetti, he swallowed his mouthful.

'If you love these kids you'll do it,' I said, gesturing at the kids, lying on their beds watching television. They were so engrossed in whatever they were watching that they hadn't heard a word I had said.

Mat nodded, wiping the pasta sauce from his mouth. 'You're right,' he said, understanding where I was coming from immediately.

'I have to drop the kids back to her tomorrow; I'll have a word while I'm there,' he said, putting down his fork and lying down next to his kids. They absentmindedly put their arms around him, still immersed in the television.

When it was time to take the kids back to Michelle the next day, Mat packed their bits and pieces up; the kids gave me a kiss and ran out to the car.

'Good luck,' I said, my heart brimming with pride.

'See you soon,' Mat replied, pecking me on the lips.

He was gone several hours. As I waited I watched Maxi's little tummy rise and fall as he slept like an angel in his cot.

When Mat returned he looked light as a feather.

'How did you go?' I asked apprehensively.

'Great, really good actually,' he said, smiling. 'I sat down with her and her boyfriend and I apologised for everything bad that

I may have done in the past to upset her. I told her she was an awesome mum and I really just wanted us to get along and be able to talk normally for the kids' sake.' Tears began to well up in my eyes.

'I am so proud of you!' I grabbed hold of him and cried with joy.

He pushed me away softly so I could see his eyes.

'You were right, Chloe, it meant so much to the kids to see us together talking normally. They were ecstatic, running around the house.' We sat together holding hands in silence for some time, contemplating the healing that would take place from this day forward.

It wasn't all fairy tales from that moment on. We still had a long way to go to mend Michelle's hurt and the pain that had spilled over into her family, but it was a start.

20

Irrational streams of blood are staining Earth …

— W.B. Yeats, 'The Gyres'

Christmas Day, 2009: Much as I adore having Christmas with my family despite the inevitable stresses, this year we decided not to travel with the kids. Instead we chose to have lunch with Mat's Aunty Teresa and Uncle Arthur, who lived on the Gold Coast at Worongary, more inland from where we lived. Such sweet, salt-of-the-earth people; Teresa reminded Mat very much of his mum, so she was definitely a safe haven for him. Jack and Skyla were with Michelle that Christmas, so we only had the two little ones with us.

It had been a year since that life-changing conversation about Max with my dad in Woy Woy. It had sent us on quite an emotional rollercoaster ride and even though it had been tough going, I was grateful for it. That confrontation had put us on the right path with Max, enabling us to unlock his true identity — now and in the future. Before I felt hopeless, but now I had hope.

The decision not to fly was a tough one. I was so used to being with my family at Christmas, and I didn't want to miss out on that feeling of being surrounded by loved ones. But although Max had been receiving intensive therapy since March, there were still plenty of trying times with him. We had had one of the most demanding years of our life, and together Mat and I decided that the stress involved in flying with Max and Phoenix was not going to be worth it for us. We wanted to relax and be in our own environment. Max was a lot more manageable when we were at home — and unpredictable when we weren't. I didn't want to burden anyone else with him.

When we arrived the house was bustling with children, all running in and out and jumping in the pool. It was a typically humid Gold Coast day, so the kids were having water bomb fights and chasing each other around with water pistols.

Max and Phoenix became very excited to see so much commotion, each in their own way. Phoenix immediately joined in with the other kids, laughing and running around. Max began flapping his arms and running around on the spot. I had come to know this as his 'stim' or self-stimulating behaviour. Many people with autism have some repetitive thing they do to deal with anxiety, excitement, fear or anger, like flapping, rocking or repeating words. (Mind you, many non-ASD people do too — if you tend to doodle, pace or twirl your hair, you're stimming.) He eventually began running after the other kids, yelling in his gobbledygook language. I don't think the other kids minded; they were all having a ball.

Mat and I sat down with the adults and chatted. It was nice to catch up with family members we could just speak to without any strain. Teresa was always happy to see us. Arthur and Teresa's house was very unpretentious and welcoming. The backyard where we were sitting had a pool that was fenced off; I knew the kids couldn't get out around the side, so I was reasonably relaxed.

I was enjoying a glass of champagne and chatting with Aunty Teresa when a blood-curdling scream came from around the side of the house. Max had been playing with a remote control car that one of the other boys was controlling. He had found it amusing to chase around after it, and the last I saw he had followed it up the side path.

Mat got up first and ran to him. I was frozen to my seat, anticipating the worst. Usually when Max hurt himself he didn't come running to be comforted, he would come running to inflict pain on me. Mat brought him around to us and my heart leapt into my throat. He had obviously fallen over and grazed his nose and his face. There was blood dripping off his nose and he was licking it with his tongue.

It is such a horrible feeling to see your son's own blood. I remember when he was a baby, cutting his finger by accident while I was trimming his nails. I was devastated then, but this was so much worse. As a mum, whenever your baby gets hurt — no matter how it happened — you always blame yourself.

The funny thing was that Max didn't seem to be anywhere near as fazed as I was about his condition. In fact he seemed not to feel it at all and was more concerned with continuing to play with the remote control car. But that was our cue to leave and that was our Christmas Day, 2009. Would it have been any more stressful to get on a plane to be with my family?

One of my missions is to make sure our kids learn how to do things for themselves. This is something that is hammered home in Max's therapy. It goes against your maternal instincts at first: from the very beginning you're trying to 'read' the needs of a baby who doesn't have words to say whether they are hungry, or hot, or tired. Even later on, you feel that it is your role to know when they are thirsty and hand them a glass of water without them asking for it, or to know what they are gesturing to in the pantry without making them say what they want.

At Little Souls, even helping a child pull their pants back up after toilet time was discouraged. The staff would rather have the child sit on the floor with one leg in their pants and one leg out, so that they would eventually learn to do the rest unassisted. All of this was about training these kids to look after themselves rather than be reliant on someone else for the rest of their lives. Let them struggle and make mistakes so they can learn what works and how best to do things for themselves. It's a principle that applies not only to Max but to all children — adults too, if it comes to it. It doesn't matter how many times you fall down with your leg stuck in your pants, the more often you do it the faster you work out how to get up again.

I could see now that I had been hindering Max's progress by doing everything for him. Once I saw it, I became enraged by my stupidity, my failure not to see this lesson from the very beginning. The one way I saw to take this rage out in a productive way was to get better. I love the saying 'Stay bitter or get better' — well, now was the time to get better. In fact, I decided that the whole family needed to sharpen up when it came to dealing with Max. I became the Therapy Cop. It got to the stage where I would not even open the door for him unless he said, 'Open door, please.' Many a cold night was spent outside our front door waiting for Max to say those three words.

Max had progressed so much with his therapy that he was able to ask for things himself spontaneously, and one step further, he could get things for himself. Now, if he was thirsty he could get himself a drink. He would go to the cupboard, get out a cup, and then pour some water from the spout in the face of our fridge.

One day I was in the laundry putting on a load of washing when I heard a loud bang and then glass shattering. I ran out to find Max standing in front of the fridge surrounded by broken glass. He must have somehow found a glass tumbler rather than the plastic cups I usually left on the bottom shelf for him. He began to take a few steps toward me, the glass crunching under his bare feet.

'Stop, Max, don't move!' I yelled. His bloodied feet kept moving, the glass audibly cracking under his feet and piercing the skin.

He began to scream. I reached down and scooped him up quickly before he could do any more damage to himself. His feet were dripping with blood; great chunks of glass were embedded deep in the soles. A primal wail reverberated through his body.

'Oh God, oh God!' I moaned, tears falling down my face. I looked into his pain-stricken face and felt a hurt deep inside my heart. I stroked his hair and rocked him back and forth as I wept. It's devastating when your child has absolutely no comprehension of what you are asking them to do or not to do. I didn't know how I was going to get the glass out of his feet without Max struggling violently. As his wails began to subside I gently lifted up his feet to assess the damage. There were two small pieces of glass in one foot and one big piece in the other. I carried him to the couch and fumbled around behind me for the remote control. I figured that if I put on his favourite show he would be less inclined to realise what was going on. I sat him down in front of SpongeBob SquarePants and proceeded to pluck shards of glass from his little feet. Bizarrely, from out of nowhere Max began singing the theme song of the show.

'Oh ... who ... lives in a pineapple under the sea?'

'SpongeBob SquarePants,' I replied as I pulled the first piece of glass from his foot.

He flinched but continued on with his version of the song.

'Yadda de yadda do yadda de yaaaa.'

'SpongeBob SquarePants.' Out came another shard of glass.

'SpongeBob SquarePants, SpongeBob SquarePants, SpongeBob.' Out with the last piece.

'SquarePants!' We finished the song together in a loud crescendo.

Max then played the pretend flute on his nose and that was the end of that debacle.

Any child can break a glass, but those everyday crises just seemed to highlight how different he was from other kids. There was a distance in the way he responded, and no sense that he was imploring me to fix the pain, as another child might. Even in pain, Max was locked away from us all.

We did — and still do — have our 'two steps back' days with Max. One sweltering day in high summer I was racing around trying to get the two kids ready to run some errands. The most important job we had to do was to take our Audi in for our changeover. Audi was a major sponsor of the Titans and because Mat was one of the team's high-profile players, they made a car available for him. Every five thousand kilometres we swapped our car for a new one, which ensured that the dealership could sell it on for a reasonable price. We had an Audi Q7, which I absolutely loved. It's the best family car — very high-tech with satellite navigation, Bluetooth and a bunch of other gadgets. It was perfect for us because it was a seven-seater, so when the older kids were with us we could fit a few friends in too.

It was a humid forty-degree day with not a puff of breeze to take the edge off. Mat was at training, like every other day. When you leave the house with two young kids you want to squeeze as much in as you can because you certainly don't want to get home only to have to go out again. What with getting two little ones in and out of car seats, it's just not worth the hassle.

Once the car was unlocked, I had a habit of strapping the kids in while still holding onto my massive bunch of keys. (So many keys — did I really need them all?) I had fastened Phoenix into her baby seat and I was struggling with Max's straps. The keyring was getting in the way, so I tossed it onto the front seat then shut Phoenix's door and walked around to the driver's door, only to find that it was locked. I tried Phoenix's door — locked. I ran to the other doors and the boot — all locked. Pressing my face up against the car window, I peered down at my keys on the front seat.

'Oh my God!' I said out loud. I must have bumped the lock button by accident. I ran to Phoenix's window. She was her usual smiley self but I could see beads of sweat beginning to form on her little brow. Glancing over at Max, I noticed he wasn't strapped in yet. I ran over to his side of the car.

'Maxi, press the button,' I said, pointing at the window button. The Q7 was so high-tech that sometimes the key just needed to be close to the ignition for the interior controls to work.

He looked at me with dazed eyes, the pupils so dilated his eyes appeared almost black.

'Press the button, c'mon, sweetheart.' I tapped on the window. He looked straight through me with a faraway glint in his eye. He seemed to have no idea what I was asking him to do; he looked totally bemused.

Phoenix began to get upset. I ran around to her window and tried to cheer her up. 'Boo!' I screamed, crouching down then jumping up to scare her. She laughed.

I decided I would have to go back inside and call Audi — they would know what to do. Thank God I hadn't already locked the house, because my mobile was inside the locked car too. I ran inside, breathing heavily. Man, it was hot!

I grabbed the cordless phone and dialled the number for information while I walked back outside to the car. 'Can you put me through to Audi on the Gold Coast, please?'

The phone began ringing. I continued to jump up and 'Boo!' the kids so they wouldn't suspect anything was wrong.

'Hello, it's Chloe Maxwell, Mat Rogers' partner. I have a bit of a situation here. My kids are locked in the car that you guys have lent us and it's getting hotter and hotter — can you please help me?' My voice was shaking with desperation.

The man took my details and assured me he was sending someone out right away. Even so, I knew they were more than thirty minutes away — a long time for two kids to be sitting in a black car in direct sunlight with the windows up.

Why couldn't Max understand me? Several weeks earlier he understood what 'push the button' meant — in fact, he could say it himself. But now when I really needed him to understand he goes blank.

As the sun continued to move higher in the cloudless sky, I kept trying to take the kids' minds off being trapped in that sauna. I'm sure if a neighbour had seen me they would have thought I was completely mad, jumping up and down and peekabooing through the closed car windows.

After fifteen minutes or so my jokes began to wear thin and the kids were beginning to look really uncomfortable. Their faces were turning crimson from the heat and they were drenched in sweat, their hair slicked to their foreheads. I spotted a half-full water bottle on the floor of the car and gestured to Max.

'Drink of water, Max, look.' Miraculously he understood me this time and got out of his seat and picked up the bottle. He took a long swallow.

'Ta for Phoenix, Max.' He hopped back in his seat and stared blankly out the window.

'Ta for Phoenix, please, Maxi. Please.' I pleaded with him for five minutes, hoping he would understand. All of a sudden he passed the bottle to her. She grabbed it and sculled the remaining water. A wave of relief swept over me; this would buy us some more time until the Audi guy arrived.

Another fifteen minutes later, an Audi TT screeched to a halt out the front of our house. A man jumped out, pointed a set of keys at the car and pushed the button. I heard the familiar click of the doors unlocking and I flung them open.

'Oh thank you! Thank you!' I exclaimed emotionally, clutching Max while undoing Phoenix's straps.

'You're welcome,' he said and with that he got back in his car and drove away.

That had to be one of the most harrowing thirty minutes I'd had for a long time. I just couldn't fathom why Max didn't understand me. I guess this was another sign to add to the growing list of symptoms that I would come to recognise as simply part of his condition. It was another crisis point that brought it home to me yet again that Max was not like the rest of us.

21

No honour leave its mighty monument,
Has but one comfort left: all triumph would
But break upon his ghostly solitude.

— W.B. Yeats, 'Thoughts Upon the Present State of the World'

Phoenix's birthday was fast approaching. I wasn't usually one for having big celebrations and parties for the kids, especially since the few I had had for Max didn't turn out the way I wanted them to. He never really understood what was going on. As children arrived and greeted him with big smiles and colourful presents, he would stare right through them with a glazed expression of mild interest on his face. Without fail there would be some disagreement or another that would end in tears because Max had cracked someone over the head with a toy or pushed them over. On his first birthday he didn't want to play with the other kids at all, but when he smacked one of them in the face he thought that was hilarious. I've still got a photo of Max and this other little girl: Max is laughing and the other one is just looking stunned. His social graces with other kids were far from well-developed, and I guess that was incredibly embarrassing for me. So I decided I wouldn't organise a party for his fourth birthday; instead my mum and grandmother flew up and we took him and Phoenix out for the day. That was enough for Max.

Phoenix, on the other hand, was incredibly social and loved the idea of having a party with her friends, so I set about arranging one for her. We went to the supermarket when Max was at kindy and chose some pretty princess invitations, lolly bags and the all-important lollies. She had a few little friends in the street I could invite but most of her friends were at Little Souls, where she now attended kindy three days a week. Her classmates there were a mixture of autistic kids and typically developed kids, and Phoenix was friends with all of them. So invitations went out to about twenty-five kids in total. Mum and grandma decided to fly up so that they could be at Phoenix's party too.

One mother in particular, Nathalia, was so overwhelmed by the invitation that she sent me a text thanking me so much for inviting her daughter Maggie to the party. Maggie was one of the ASD kids at the centre. She was three and a half and had never been invited to a party before. Nathalia told me she had cried when she read the invitation. Little things we take for granted, such as our child being invited to a birthday party, are massive milestones to the parents of an ASD child.

With such a big group, we planned to hold the party at Laguna Park in Palm Beach, one of the best parks for kids around and not too far from us. But a few days before the party the forecast was for torrential rain, so I made a snap decision to change the location to an indoor play centre in Southport instead. I had been to a party there once before and I thought it would be really fun for all of the kids.

Around this time, I had started doing some work on *The Matty Johns Show*, which had just kicked off on Channel Seven. Matty was a colourful ex-football player who was best known for the characters he played on Channel Nine's *The Footy Show*. Unfortunately he got himself into a spot of bother that was, I believed, really an issue for him and his wife to resolve but was dragged out into the spotlight by the media. The matter was resolved, but due to the media attention Matty lost his job. The media being a cutthroat and opportunistic world, Channel Seven picked Matty up and gave him his own show. Many thought it would fail — in fact many hoped it would, but Matty was proving the critics wrong.

A few days before the party I got a call from the producers asking me if I could do a red carpet interview with Hollywood teen heart-throb Zac Efron on the same day as the party. I calculated that I could fly to Sydney for the interview straight after the party, as it was only meant to go for two hours. I would need to have my makeup done and ready for when I arrived at the studio, though, so I enlisted the help of a friend Jodie-Lee Gheoghan.

Party day rolled around, and at seven am I was on the balcony getting my hair and makeup done for television, hoping that the neighbours wouldn't think I was going to all this trouble for a three-year-old's party. When we arrived at the play centre I felt rather out-of-place with my caked-on makeup, especially when the other mothers arrived looking very casual indeed. I lost track of how many times I excused my appearance that day. I didn't usually wear makeup at all for kindy pickup and dropoff, so I figured I should explain the sudden change!

Parents streamed in to the play centre, dragged by excited children. The shrieks and squeals were deafening. As I looked around the throng of kids going wild, I spotted Phoenix and Max on a big jumping castle shaped like a shark. They were peering through the mouth with its inflated teeth, holding hands and jumping. They were having so much fun.

A wall of mazes and staircases and slippery dips lined the other side of the centre, and beyond that was a ball pit. Four or five boys were going absolutely nuts in there, slamming into each other and laughing. I decided Phoenix and Max probably shouldn't go in the ball pit today.

It was obvious who the ASD kids were, aside from Max, as most of them only wanted to go in the fenced-off baby area. They were overwhelmed by the colours and the noise and all the other kids.

I walked into the baby area, where there was a selection of little cars, beanbags and a play boat. One of the ASD boys from Little Souls, James, and his mum Di were there. James was refusing to get off a piece of equipment; he kept looking at a mural on the wall then cowering in fear. Di was always so lovely to talk to at kindy and we had both comforted each other at different times in the reception room of Little Souls when our boys were proving to be too much.

'Hi, Di, how are you?' I asked, trying to sound upbeat. I could see the stress lines forming on her face.

'OK, you know,' she said, a pained smile playing across her face.

'What's up, James?' I asked, rhetorically, of course. James was a little bit older than Max and had no speech at all. I always tried to engage with the ASD kids, even though I knew they would not engage back. I didn't want their parents to see me treating their kids differently to others.

'He's OK, he's just a little overwhelmed,' Di replied for him, as us ASD mums do. 'He plays on this same piece of equipment at kindy, so he's familiar with it. He's scared of the face that's painted on the wall though.' She gestured up at a big cartoon drawing of a face.

'I don't think he realises it's just a painting,' she offered, staring up at the mural.

Suddenly high-pitched screaming interrupted our conversation. I turned around to see Nathalia behind us, struggling with her daughter Maggie. The same Nathalia who was so excited her daughter had finally been invited to a birthday party that she cried.

'Hi, Nathalia; hi, Maggie,' I said, trying to feign indifference to the noise coming from the little girl. She was screaming so hard that her face had turned crimson and the veins were popping out of her neck. Nathalia and I tried in vain to distract her with different toys. It just would not work. I could tell Nathalia was trying to stay calm even though she was absolutely devastated inside. It was heartbreaking: she had been so looking forward to her daughter doing something normal for a change. They had been there only ten minutes when Nathalia had to decide that it was too much. She made their farewells regretfully and left.

I chased after Nathalia to give her Maggie's lolly bag. 'Are you going to be OK?'

'Yes, it's just upsetting, that's all,' she replied as the tears began to roll down her cheeks. Maggie was still screaming as Nathalia took her hand and led her across to their car.

I headed back inside, stopping by the table laden with food and lollies to make sure Mum and Grandma were OK. Grandma had hearing aids and I wasn't sure she was coping with all of the noise.

'What was wrong with that little one?' Grandma asked as I came across. She absolutely loved kids and hated to see any of them upset.

'She's autistic and this is the first-ever party she has been to. It was just too overwhelming for her,' I had to explain. I told Mum and Grandma about how excited the mum had been as her daughter had never been invited to a party before; as I explained, they both got very emotional.

I think Mum and Grandma were beginning to understand the difference now between autistic kids and typically developed kids. Up until then I suspect they had been hanging onto the hope that this was all just some misunderstanding and Max was fine. My grandma is eighty years old and autism was not something that people talked about when she was growing up. People who were different were just labelled 'retards' and hidden away from the rest of society, so there wasn't a whole lot of awareness in her age group of what this diagnosis could mean. The incidence of autism is increasing year on year, so that now around one in a hundred and ten children are on the spectrum. That can mean that many older people become hardened and almost cynical about an ASD diagnosis. I don't think Mum and Grandma were any exception. Although Mum acknowledges the condition in general, to this day she has never once suggested that there is anything unusual about Max. I suspect she thinks that we're all quite mad and he will be fine. Max was her first grandson, so he is special to her in that respect. Like me, my mum must have conjured up 'future memories' — dreams and aspirations for Max that may never take place. It is never easy to bury those dreams.

I had to leave the party early to go to my interview, but on the way to the airport I made sure I texted Nathalia. I wanted her to know that Max was the same in the beginning and not to worry — Maggie would definitely be invited again. Parents of ASD kids often said to me that once their child had acted out of turn at a friend's house or a party, they were not invited back again. Because the child was simply not able to interact properly with other children they were excluded from those relationships, which was the opposite of what they really needed.

It had been a while since I had done any real television. My stint on *It Takes Two* was two years back. I'd done some radio work and some bits and pieces for the *20 to 1* show, but it was all pretty easy stuff. For *20 to 1* I was filmed chatting about various pop culture topics once a month. I just had to travel up to Channel Ten at Mount Coot-tha, on the west side of Brisbane, so I didn't even have to leave Queensland.

It had suited me during that time, because I had been consumed with motherhood. Raising Max with his special needs, as well as Phoenix along with Jack who was living with us full-time and Skyla part-time, left very little time to pursue anything else. But now that Max was settled quite nicely into his therapy routine, I was feeling more and more confident that I could tackle a new challenge. Since Mat had announced his retirement I figured I needed to get back out there again to help out financially.

More than anything, though, I wanted to get back into television. It really was my passion. I love to entertain, and the sheer adrenalin rush of live television appeals to my nature.

The opportunity came up for me to be a guest on *The Matty Johns Show*, so I flew down to Sydney on the morning of the show. I was to be in a segment called 'Are you smarter than a footballer?' A footballer, another celebrity and I would be asked a series of trivia questions, and the winner would score a gift basket with an assortment of prizes from various sponsors. It sounded like an easy gig, one that I could have some fun with.

I was up against actor Gary Sweet and NRL player Eric Grothe Junior. Gary Sweet may have ended up winning the competition, but I ended up getting a regular gig out of that little appearance. The producers liked me so much they requested I do an interview for the next show with the stars of Nitro Circus, Travis Pastrana and Jolene Van Vugt. I knew quite a bit about the show as it was one of Mat's favourite TV shows at the time — Travis and his mates get about the world riding dirt bikes, base-jumping and performing a bunch of crazy stunts. They were in town to film a show, so I headed out to Homebush Stadium to speak to the guys.

One thing I had mentioned to the producers at my last appearance was that I was up for anything. Once they told me what they had in mind for me, I regretted that statement instantly. Too late for regrets, though.

'OK, Chloe, after you finish the interview, you'll be standing here and Travis is going to do a back flip over your head,' my producer Sandra began explaining.

'I'm sorry — a what over my what?' I was a touch nervous about the interview itself, let alone potentially copping a motorcycle in the head. I really wanted this job though.

'Never mind, I'm good. Let's do it!' Travis and Jolene were heading towards me, up to the top of the giant ramp where we would be doing our interview.

I worded them up on what some of my questions might be; I even told Jolene to say she thought Matty Rogers was hot so that I could use the humorous comeback that I had ready. On air I said something like, 'Watch it, girlfriend, or you'll be doing a back flip without a bike in a minute!' I thought this was hilarious but she was clearly unimpressed.

The interview was over; now it was time for the stunt. I stood there with waves of terror running through me. I began to speak; to this day I have no idea what I said as a motorbike went flying above my head.

'I think I need to go change my pants now,' was my closing remark as I walked off-screen.

When we got back to the studio, everyone said the segment went down really well, so I was booked in to do some more entertainment interviews. My next interview would be with Usher.

I was a big fan of his music and had interviewed him once before, many years ago with Channel V, but I had not been in the music zone for a good while. I could sing you the theme song for *Dora the Explorer* or *SpongeBob SquarePants* without even blinking, but Usher was a serious musician. I, however, am not a serious interviewer, so I set out to do an interview with him that would be different to the thousand other interviews he would have done while he was in Australia.

Usher was doing a press junket, so there were reporters from every major media outlet lined up to interview him in the Sebel Hotel in Sydney. In a junket, the star's management book out a set of rooms in a hotel; the star hops from room to room, doing interviews all day long. It can be extremely tedious for the artist and incredibly repetitive, as they get asked the same questions over and over again.

With the help of my producer Sandra, I had come up with a few questions that we hoped would be entertaining for our viewers — and for Usher, too. We set up the lighting, chairs and camera in our allocated room, then waited for Usher to be finished next door. All of a sudden a large dark man appeared at the door. It was Usher's bodyguard, closely followed by the man himself.

My cameraman had brought his daughter especially for her to get an autograph and she was squirming with delight in the corner as Usher walked into the room. I stood up to shake his hand and found myself towering over him.

The interview went really well, especially when I asked about his kids.

'Are you a hands-on dad with your kids?' I asked.

'Of course,' Usher replied.

'Do you change diapers?' I asked cheekily as he adjusted his dark glasses.

'Of course.'

'Have you had a diaper explosion?'

'Yeah, a yellow one. It just shot up,' he said as we both erupted into laughter. Nothing like a poo joke to break the ice.

I ended the interview by asking Usher if I could try tackling him — this was a football show, after all.

'You mean you want to tackle me right now?' he asked.

'Where's that big bodyguard of yours?' I asked.

'He's gone,' Usher replied as I passed him the ball and ran at him. I actually put a hit on Usher — a pretty weak one I admit, but it made for good television and once again my producers were happy.

I spent a few months travelling back and forth to Sydney, interviewing stars and bands such as Richard Branson, Russell Brand, Harry Kewell, Train, 30 Seconds to Mars — I even flew to the States to interview Kelly Rowland from Destiny's Child. I was back, baby.

Looking back at everything I went through with Max, I would never have predicted we would get through all of that the way we did, nor that I might end up back where I had. From this I learned that when things look their bleakest, know and trust that it will get better. They do say that the worst time to judge anything is when you are at your lowest. When you're looking up from way down there, it's hard to get your perspective right.

The Matty Johns Show only lasted a season before it was canned following a dispute over scheduling, but I had my mojo again and nothing would stop me now. The more challenges I overcame in life and the more I forced myself outside my comfort zone, the stronger I became.

22

A starlit or a moonlit dome disdains
All that man is,
All mere complexities,
The fury and the mire of human veins.

— W.B. Yeats, 'Byzantium'

Every now and then when Mat would get a day off training he would take care of the kids in the morning so I could enjoy a sleep-in. He usually only had one day off a week, so these rare occasions were a real luxury.

On one of these mornings the kids were up particularly early. Mat arose to switch on their cartoons and get them their bottles. Our kids both loved their 'bottle hot' as they called it. They've gotten over that phase now, but it was close to an obsession for both of them for quite some time.

Gratefully I turned over and went back to sleep with the familiar sounds of *Tom and Jerry* filtering through from the living room. Just as I was drifting into a blissful half-dream about Mat being at home full-time one day, my reverie was pierced by

Maxi's screams. I sat bolt upright in bed, straining to discern what was going on out there. I could hear Mat's voice trying to pacify him but Max was clearly terribly upset; his screams became more shrill with every calm word.

'Here's your bottle, Max,' Mat was saying in a soothing voice. He was always so incredibly calm in these situations. He never failed to impress me — what had I done to deserve someone so patient and loving? God knows patience was never one of my virtues. More often than not I would lose my temper at times like this. It's very difficult to help a child in obvious distress when they can't tell you what is wrong. You can't stop your child crying and you feel like a failure as a parent.

'What's wrong, Maxi?' Once more I could hear that patient, loving voice. Max screamed again.

'Darling?' I croaked from the bedroom. I thought I might know what the problem was.

'Are you trying to give Max a pink bottle, by any chance?' I asked.

'Yeah,' Mat responded. 'How did you know?'

'He won't eat or drink out of anything that's pink. He knows that's not his colour, it's Phoenix's,' I explained matter-of-factly.

The screams died down; Mat had obviously swapped the bottles over. I rolled over onto my side in bed and stared at the framed photographs on my dresser. I contemplated the photos of Mat and me at the Titans ball, the kids, my brother and Kate on their wedding day. I wondered how families with an ASD child coped when both parents had to go to work. Without the strongest lines of communication, it would be near impossible for two working adults who spend five days a week at work to have any semblance of a happy life with an ASD child.

I felt so lucky to be able to spend so much time with my special boy so that I could understand him so well. I was beginning to recognise my son's little quirks — and I was determined that was how they would remain, as quirks. I believe we all have them. Over the years most of us simply become better at hiding them.

Skyla was born with very cute 'sticky-outy ears'. At least, they were cute when she was little, but as she began to mature she became terribly self-conscious about them.

One day Skyla said to me, 'Chloe, I hate my ears.'

'Why, sweetie?' I asked, already knowing what that answer would be.

'I get really teased about them at school. The boys are so mean to me.' My heart broke as little tears traced their way down her sun-kissed cheeks. She had the most piercing blue eyes, one of which had a little freckle in it.

Kids can be very cruel in the playground. I had experienced that firsthand and I had no desire for Skyla to be subjected to the same treatment. I would never forgive myself if she had to go through what my sister had at the hands of bullies.

If other children were tormenting this pretty little thing about her ears, I wondered how they would react to Max. There was no doubt that he would have to face bullying eventually, but I really didn't know how I would cope with that. I suspected I'd want to go and tan their backsides.

The decision was made that Skyla would get her ears pinned. It was a relatively uncomplicated procedure that would just mean one morning in day surgery. She wouldn't be able to run around for several weeks, though, and she would have a bandage around her head for a little while. We decided the school holidays would be a good time to do it.

Mat took her to the hospital in the morning and waited with her while her anaesthetic took effect; Skyla had never had surgery before and she was very scared. After her little eyes closed, Mat left for training. He would still be in training when she came out, so it was up to me to pick her up.

I didn't have anyone to mind the kids, so I had to take Max and Phoenix with me. We parked in the car park under the hospital and I popped Phoenix in her pram and held Max's hand as we walked across to the lift.

Like most young kids, Max was absolutely fascinated with lifts and always wanted to press all of the buttons. We hopped in happily and Max pressed the button for our floor. When the lift doors opened, I began to push Phoenix out in her pram. Max, however, was reluctant to get out all of a sudden.

'Come on, Maxi, let's go,' I said in an enthusiastic voice, as though we were headed for somewhere really fun. He held tight to the railing with his head lowered and looked up at me, his brow furrowed. I reversed the pram quickly, grabbed his hand and yanked him out of the lift. He began to cry. Frightened by my yanking movement and Max's howling, Phoenix began to cry too.

We entered the hushed waiting room, where several people waited quietly and a sign encouraged people to turn off their mobile phones, clearly to ensure a peaceful atmosphere for the patients in recovery.

Every head turned as the scream train rolled in.

A well-groomed lady looked with disdain over the newspaper she was reading. I cast daggers at her with one look and she went back to reading her paper. In those situations I sometimes hope that the person will say something, just so that I can verbally tear shreds off someone. I don't know if that would make me feel better but I suspect it might go some way to helping.

I walked over to the receptionist, who was doing a very bad job of pretending the noise wasn't bothering her.

'Hello, I'm here to pick up Skyla Rogers from day surgery,' I said, also feigning indifference to the noise.

The woman tapped a few keys on her computer, her long fake red nails clicking loudly.

'She's not quite ready to go yet, she's still unconscious. You'll have to wait twenty minutes or so. Take a seat,' she said, gesturing to the waiting room. An audible sigh rippled around the occupants when they realised we were going to be with them for a while longer.

I gave the kids some chips to eat in an attempt to keep them quiet, but this didn't help at all. Max was still fascinated with the lift and kept trying to escape back out to it every few minutes.

A nurse brought in some colouring pencils and paper. 'Here you go,' she said compassionately, giving me a little nod of understanding. She obviously had kids or at least knew how to entertain them. Phoenix was interested in them, but Max picked up the pencils and threw them across the room.

'OK, let's go see the lift,' I said, accepting the fact that he was not going to be diverted by some pencils and paper.

We went back out into the foyer and I let the kids run around chasing each other. I could see people in the other wards looking at me through the glass, no doubt wondering why I was letting my wild children run loose in the hospital. As long as they weren't screaming I didn't care. Suddenly the lift opened; a group of people came out of it and started walking towards us. There were so many that I grabbed Phoenix by the hand and moved out of their way. After they had dispersed I looked for Max. He was nowhere to be seen.

I ran up and down the corridor, calling his name. 'Max — Maxi!

'Oh my God,' I murmured, realising what had happened.

'Are you OK, sweetie?' the kind nurse who had given us the colouring pencils asked, seeing me clearly in distress.

'My son ... I ... I think he went into the lift,' I said frantically.

Running to the glass atrium in the middle of the building, I looked down at the many floors of the hospital below. Clutching Phoenix's hand tight I then turned my head and looked up at the many floors above. I began to sweat. This was a big building — he could be anywhere.

'What's his name, sweetie?' she asked as some hospital staff began to gather around.

'His name is Max … but … oh, God! He's autistic but doesn't always answer to his name.' My voice was wild and shaky.

The employees began combing the halls and several of them got in the lift. 'Wait here,' the kind woman said. 'In case he comes back.'

I nodded, tears welling in my eyes. Sensing my unease, Phoenix began to cry too. I strapped her back into her pram so I knew that at least she would be safe and I pushed her up and down the hallway. I paced back and forth, praying that they would find him. Pressing my face to the window I looked down to the entrance, half expecting to see him wander out onto the main road. Every time the lift bell went I ran and stood there, hoping to see his face. Instead patients, doctors and nurses came out of the lift and eyed me suspiciously when I didn't get in.

Finally, exhausted with worry, I collapsed in a heap on the floor next to Phoenix's pram. The lady with the red fake fingernails came out and saw me in a crumpled heap on the floor.

'Skyla is now ready to be escorted home,' she said, looking me over as though I had the plague.

'OK, thank you. I've just lost my son in the lift, there are some people trying to find him for me right now,' I said, realising the absurdity of what I just said and getting annoyed with this woman for making me say it.

'OK, well, when you're ready let me know,' she replied with an amused look on her face.

'Oh, I'll let you know,' I mumbled angrily under my breath.

The elevator buzzed and the kind lady emerged. She was holding Max's hand.

'Oh, Maxi ... Where have you been?' I asked, running to him and embracing him tightly. I was so relieved.

'Thank you so much,' I said. 'Where was he?'

'He was wandering around on the fourth floor; one of the orderlies found him,' she replied. 'He'll be alright now. Do you need any more help?' she asked.

'No, thank you, thank you so much.' I was so grateful and so relieved we could now get Skyla and get the hell out of here.

I pushed Phoenix's pram back into the waiting room, clutching Max's hand so tight I could have wrenched it right off. Red fingernail lady gestured to the right of the counter. 'Just go around to the right there and you'll see her.' She barely looked up from the computer as we passed.

We walked into a big room where quite a few patients were recovering. At the end of the room there was Skyla, lying in a hospital bed. Her head was wrapped in a big bandage. She looked very drowsy still.

'Hi, Chloe,' she said in a croaky little voice.

'Hello, sweetie. Are you ready to go?' I asked, pretending nothing had happened.

'Yeah, I want to go home now,' she replied, slowly getting up off the bed.

'Me too, Bub. Me too.'

23

The Soul. Seek out reality, leave things that seem.
The Heart. What, be a singer born and lack a theme?

— W.B. Yeats, 'Vacillation'

For us, our first fundraising weekend was not just any event: it was our opportunity to introduce 4 ASD Kids to the world and to make sure it started its life with a bang. It had all come together in just over six weeks — a miracle in its own right, as anyone who has ever organised a public event will know. We had taken a major gamble putting our name to an event with so little time to organise it, but several frenetic weeks of activity had paid off. It was the weekend before Christmas and our 4 ASD Kids charity weekend was upon us.

We had hit the phone hard in the lead-up, ringing people and asking them to buy weekend packages or tables to individual events, or to donate items for auction. Not just any old thing, either: we wanted money-can't-buy auction items. Mat was absolutely amazing at drumming up support. The way he sees it, if he's putting his name to something, then he has to do everything he can to ensure it's a success. That's the mindset that makes him so successful in life.

In the midst of our final preparations for our big 4 ASD Kids fundraising weekend, we got a call from our lawyer, Ashleigh. He was adamant that we needed to meet another of his clients, a successful entrepreneur called Chris. Ashleigh told Mat that Chris had two autistic kids, and was keen to support our charity in any way he could. Apparently Chris and his wife had seen our interview on television and were determined to meet us and help us.

Ashleigh picked Mat up the following day and they headed down to Lennox Head, a beautiful beach town an hour's drive south. Chris and his wife and their kids lived there in a stunning home on a couple of acres not far from the beach. Driving through Lennox Head took Mat back to his youth: this was where he spent a great part of his childhood. His parents had owned the pub on the beach there and he had spent many days surfing the breaks at Lennox Beach.

I'm not quite sure what went on there that day, but Mat came back full of praise for Chris and his family and bearing a case of Grange Hermitage signed by Bill Clinton. I was blown away: this guy had given us a case of one of the most revered wines you can lay hands on — signed by a former president of the United States, no less — so that we could auction it to raise money that would give kids access to early intervention programs. These people were clearly passionate about the cause. They had also invited our whole family to come down and visit next time. They especially wanted to meet our Max.

The day we drove down to Lennox Head I really didn't know what to expect. Mat had said that they were amazing people but I wasn't prepared for just how inspirational and life changing our meeting would be.

We pulled into a driveway surrounded by perfectly manicured gardens, in the midst of which nestled a Colonial-style mansion. Immediately smiling kids began to appear from the side of the house, followed by Chris and Jeanagh. They looked like the perfect family as they stood with their arms around each other, waiting excitedly for us to get out of the car. One of the three boys was feverishly bouncing a ball with a coat hanger on the pavement. He had a massive smile on his face as he observed us out of the corner of his eye.

We walked together to greet them. 'Darling, this is Chris and Jeanagh.' Mat gestured to the smiling couple.

'Hello,' I said, immediately feeling a sense of being totally welcome and at ease, even though we had only just met that minute.

'This is Sam,' said Chris, indicating the boy who had been bouncing the ball. 'He's our eldest — he's ten.'

The boy grunted excitedly and then bounded into the house ahead of us, clutching his coathanger and ball. I glimpsed the top of a nappy protruding above his board shorts.

'This is Patrick; Patrick, you remember Mat? This is his wife Chloe.' Chris tapped his son lovingly on the arm.

'Yes, hello,' the boy replied shyly.

'And this is Christopher,' Jeanagh said, pulling the seemingly distracted boy close.

'Who's this? What's your name?' Christopher said, gesturing at me.

'My name's Chloe,' I answered with a warm smile.

The little boy began writing in the air with his index finger. 'And when's your birthday?' he asked, almost absently.

'July the sixth,' I replied. Again he wrote in the air with his finger.

'Chloe, July the sixth — got it,' he said, and turned and walked away.

I looked after him quizzically as Jeanagh took me aside.

'He won't ever forget your name now,' she said. 'He writes it in the air so he can visualise — it's his way of remembering things.'

'Wow!' I said, struck by the complete contrast between Christopher and his older brother Sam.

We headed into the house, which enormous yet beautifully designed. Mat, the kids and I followed our hosts through a side door that led through the laundry. On the left were shelves and shelves full of shoes. There were a lot of feet in this house, that was for sure. We went on through another door, which led into the lounge room. The walls were lined with drawings of the house itself, and there were countless family photos and pictures of the boys everywhere. I noticed a beautiful picture of all of them on the trampoline. They looked so happy and — well, normal.

I was instantly drawn to this family and everything they stood for. I began to feel an inner strength growing in the pit of my stomach. It was almost as though being around these people was giving me a new fortitude in the face of my own struggles with Max, which paled in comparison to what they must face with two boys on the spectrum.

Sam, in particular, seemed to need a lot of attention. I believed Christopher to be a savant, which is one extreme on the autism spectrum. He showed all the signs of being a genius, whereas his older brother had no speech at all. This, of course, didn't mean Sam had no intellect, he simply couldn't communicate it. Too often people believe lack of communication means lack of intellect. A great example is the now-famous Carly Fleishmann, who could not communicate until the age of eleven, when she began typing her feelings on a computer.

I was so grateful these people had invited us into their house; I knew we would be friends for a long time. They would be the sort of people we could call at any time to catch up, no matter how long it had been since the last time. They more than understood where we were at and their laidback, easygoing attitude to everything was an incredible source of inspiration to me.

* * *

In the lead-up to our fundraising event, I had gone to Little Souls and filmed some of the families there so we could put together a video package to encourage people to donate. I had arranged to speak to just a few of the families, to give the audience some idea of the hardships all of these families faced financially, as well as the benefits of attending a school like Little Souls.

One couple I particularly wanted to film was Brett and Kerry Vaughan. They had two boys at Little Souls plus twins at home. Every day they travelled to Little Souls from Tweed Heads, a drive of about forty kilometres each way. Robyn, the founder of Little Souls, had told me they were dipping into their superannuation fund in order to afford therapy for their boys. I had often noticed them at the centre, helping out where they could. They were one family that especially touched my heart: they were doing it tough, yet they were giving so much to help other families. Mat and I and the other 4 ASD Kids organisers had decided that Brett and Kerry's two boys would be the first to benefit from the money we raised. They didn't know that yet.

I cried pretty much the whole time we were filming. I was trying to ask very emotional questions — I guess my time on *The X Factor* was coming in handy for something. I figured if I was crying, our guests would be crying on the night too — hopefully while also writing big cheques.

These families' stories were heartbreaking enough without

any need to dramatise things. Each of them was so inspirational: they maintained such a positive outlook despite the enormous challenges they faced every single day. These people were your classic Aussie battlers, trying to give their special needs kids the best opportunity for a normal life. It was not only sheer hard work, it was also an enormously expensive exercise, and for each family the cost in terms of time and money was massive.

The weekend kicked off with a golf day at Links Hope Island resort. Hundreds of people had paid a fee to play in the competition, and Mat was driven around in a buggy to have a hit with each group. The day went off really well, and was followed by a welcome cocktail party at the Hyatt at Sanctuary Cove — the very same place we had celebrated our wedding.

Awards were given for different categories in the golf, then we were treated to some stunning opera with Melinda Schneider and Lachlan Baker. As the music finished, the most amazing fireworks lit up the sky. I was standing there, champagne in hand, full of excitement for what the weekend would bring. I had barely sipped it when Mat and I were called up to the stage to say a few words.

I had not spoken to Mat yet that evening, as he had been doing a live cross for the news on the other side of the party. Looking over as I started towards the stage, I saw him making his way through the crowd. We stepped up onstage almost simultaneously and each took a microphone, staring out at the massive crowd in front of us.

'Welcome, everybody, to the inaugural 4 ASD Kids charity weekend,' I began. 'We are so grateful that you are all here. Our son Max was diagnosed with autism at the beginning of this year and we have seen firsthand the benefits that intensive early intervention can have. We have also seen the price tag that therapy can come with.' I gulped hard, fighting back the emotion.

'Max has come so far in such a short period of time, we thought everyone should have access to this therapy. Everyone does — but the one problem is money. It's very expensive for these kids to get the care they need. We decided to help those who cannot afford treatment.' I handed over to Mat.

'This weekend is about coming together and pooling our resources to help these kids and their families.' I looked over at Mat to see his green eyes filling with tears, but he continued. 'True greatness is not just being great at something. It's using what you are great at to help others and that's what we should all aim to do this weekend. There are still some spots available for our other events over the weekend, so come along, bring some friends and dig deep. Thank you.'

We held hands as we left the stage, nervous but excited at the prospect of what this weekend could mean to so many.

Everyone was then ushered over to the Woolshed for music and dancing. Far from the rustic shed that its name suggests, it's a stunning function area that lies at the bottom of an ornate staircase; inside the room was decorated with glittering stars, and the stage was set for entertainment. We partied into the early hours of the next morning to Mark Gable (ex-lead singer of the Choirboys), Paulini (one of *Australian Idol*'s best-known contestants), Casey Barnes (another *Australian Idol* discovery), and a personal favourite for Mat and me, the talented singer Danny Fai Fai.

Jack and Skyla had an absolute ball, as did the rest of the guests. We had arranged for a babysitter to mind Max and Phoenix, though the kids did join us onstage at one point, on Sunday at the Christmas carols. I was so proud of Max: up there in front of all those people he got on the microphone, and when asked what his name was, said in a lovely big voice, 'Max.' Mind you, that was after standing prominently mid-stage and rattling away in his mumbo-jumbo language. Phoenix also showed her true personality: when Sandra Sully, newsreader and one of the MCs for the event, got her in front of the microphone and asked her if she was enjoying herself, here's what she had to say: 'Go away.' That's my girl.

Saturday night's gala dinner was where we were hoping to make the most money. We had pulled every string we could think of to get auction items and we had some fantastic one-of-a-kind things that we were hoping would enable us to raise enough money to sponsor two children for a year of therapy.

The lights dimmed and on the screen above the stage, the footage from our interview with Danny Weidler began. All of the guests who had been chattering away fell silent. At its conclusion, newsreader Tim Webster — our MC, along with Sandra Sully — stepped onto the stage. He took the microphone and began the evening by welcoming everyone, then introduced the first of several special guests for the evening.

'I'd like to welcome Ben to the stage,' Tim said and looked around. 'Ben, come on down.'

Through the crowd came a teenage boy looking very dapper in a tuxedo, complete with bow tie. Close behind him was his mum, Robyn Hawkins, the founder of Little Souls Taking Big Steps.

'Welcome Ben and mum Robyn.' Tim gestured for them to speak into the microphone.

'Hello,' Ben said, a little too loudly. He began to pace around the stage.

'Now, just a bit of background on Ben,' Tim said. 'He lives with an autism spectrum disorder; however, due to benefiting from early intervention from his mother herself, he is a pretty cool guy. In fact he knows more about trains than anyone I know.' Ben now had his back to the audience; his mum Robyn tried to coerce him into turning around and facing everyone.

'Now, Ben, tell us some interesting facts about trains,' Tim asked.

Ben rose to the occasion with remarkable poise, talking about different railway lines in Australia and all around the world. Listening to him speak stirred some powerful feelings in me. When you have an ASD child, you often wonder if they will ever grow up to be able to communicate on a normal level with people. Ben gave me so much hope for the future.

After Ben finished speaking, we ran the video showing some of the families from Little Souls. There was not a dry eye in the house as these parents spoke from the heart about their kids and the difference that early intervention therapy can make.

As the video ended I walked up to the stage. Under my breath I was muttering to myself to hold it together, as my emotions were running very high.

'Good evening, everyone. I would like to welcome a couple to the stage now who you will recognise from that video, to share a little bit more with all of us.' Mat and I and the other organisers had decided to do something quite special at this stage of the evening.

'Brett and Kerry Vaughan, would you come to the stage please?' I watched with anticipation as they made their way through the crowd.

Brett and Kerry joined me onstage and I asked them a few questions about how Little Souls had helped their two boys and what the financial cost meant for them. Looking out at the crowd as Brett and Kerry spoke, I could see many people looked shocked at the hard road this lovely couple had endured. Then I dropped the big one on them.

'Despite your incredibly positive attitude, we know how hard you guys have it. And it is because of this that your boys will be the very first recipients of support from 4 ASD Kids — their therapy for next year will be fully paid for. Surprise!' The crowd erupted into applause and cheers as Brett and Kerry stood there, dumbfounded by what had just happened.

'Thank you, thank you so much,' Brett managed to stammer before they left the stage in a state of shock. I don't think they could believe what was happening. Having the cost of therapy for both boys looked after for a year would remove a massive amount of stress from this amazing family.

Right from the start, I loved what we were able to do through 4 ASD Kids. The feeling of helping someone like this far outweighed the thrill I got from a big cheque in our hands at the end of the month, or any interview with Usher or Richard Branson. I had discovered my meaning, my path for life. I was hooked.

We went on to raise more than $175,000 that evening, which meant we could help another two children. With great difficulty we chose two more kids to sponsor for therapy at Little Souls; Robyn had the pleasure of calling their families on Christmas Eve to give them the good news. I like to think it was the best Christmas present ever for them — and for Robyn, and for Mat and me too.

24

A company of friends, a conscience set at ease,
It had but made us pine the more. The abstract joy,
The half-read wisdom of daemonic images,
Suffice the ageing man as once the growing boy.

— W.B. Yeats, 'Meditations in Time of Civil War'

Max doesn't see people, he sees through people. It is as if he and I are in a bubble, floating around together. He acknowledges his family and people he knows well. Others are invisible to him. At the park, children come up wanting to engage with him; he walks right by as if they are ghosts. Often he simply stares off into nothingness, as if he is in an eternal reverie.

Apparently the human face is too complex for autistic people to comprehend. They are not aware when someone is angry, sad, hurt or even happy. When I raised my voice to Max he would simply mimic me with the same raised voice. If I was upset he would never feel the need to comfort me, which is instinctive to most humans.

At first I saw all of these attributes as the traits of a difficult child. Looking back now, I feel ashamed of the anger I felt at Max's apparent defiance.

One day Mat and I took all four kids to Robina Town Centre, a big shopping complex ten minutes drive from our home. Max and Phoenix loved the play gym area near the restaurants and cafés, so we would take a break from shopping and have a meal there so they could play where we could see them. This particular day we had asked Jack, then thirteen years old, to keep an eye on them inside the play area while Mat, Skyla and I finished our lunch. Jack is so good with Max: he carries him around and gives him big sloppy kisses, which is pretty cool for a teenager. Even knowing Jack was watching the kids, I glanced that way often to see if the kids were doing OK. Just as my eyes flicked to the top of the play equipment, they locked on Maxi standing right at the top. He had dropped his pants and commenced urinating on all of the kids below him.

I looked on in horror as small children slowly came to the realisation that the liquid coming from the sky was not in fact rain but 'wee'. Mothers ran screaming from all directions to scoop their children up and stare at the brat of a child standing above them all. Furiously they looked around for the owners of the brat while clutching their urine-soaked kids to their bosoms. Jack took off faster than I have ever seen him flee from the scene of any crime. He was just a streak of blond hair flashing across the playground.

I tapped Mat on the shoulder, interrupting his conversation with Skyla.

'What is it, darling?' he asked, slightly irritated that I had cut in on their chat and was now just sitting there mutely.

My hand was covering my mouth in shock. All I could do was point and say, 'Max.'

Mat looked up to see his son atop the highest piece of equipment in the play gym with his pants around his ankles and a big yellow stream still gushing forth.

'You better go get him, darling,' I said, recovering my voice.

'I'm not going over there,' he said resolutely.

Why is it that women seem better able to deal with humiliation than men? It was up to me, it seemed. I stood up and strode purposefully across to my little perpetrator. As I walked across I could sense eyes boring in to the back of my head: all of the people who had been enjoying their lunch now knew that there was a commotion in the play gym. Looking up, I could see Max expelling the last drops from his bladder. Distraught mothers stared at me as I opened the gate and walked over to the play gym. The playground was utterly silent.

'Pants on, Max, time to go,' I said, trying to sound like I had everything under control.

I looked over at a mother clutching a urine-soaked little girl. Her face was distorted as if she had swallowed a mouthful.

'Disgusting!' she hissed under her breath. My blood boiled as Maxi slipped his little hand into mine and looked around with his big dazed smile, as though the little man had no idea what had just taken place.

'Should I say something or just let it go?' I thought to myself. I looked back; the woman was still shaking her head at us. I turned on my heel and marched up to her.

'My son is autistic, he doesn't know that what he was doing was wrong. I'm sorry!'

'Oh — I'm sorry,' she exclaimed, her tone instantly changing from disgust to sympathy.

With that we stormed out of the playground. Mat and the kids had already gathered up our stuff and paid the bill. We walked out holding hands and we did not look back.

Mat and I had been thinking a lot about what the next year might bring. His contract with the Titans was up for renewal at the end of the year and coach John Cartwright had insinuated that there might not be a place for him at the club after that. The salary cap wouldn't allow for him to stay on with the younger talent they were hoping to bring in.

At the time, Mat was the second oldest player in the competition, next to Adam MacDougall who played for the Newcastle Knights. Mat was never one to whinge about injuries but I knew he was in constant pain every day. He would never say anything — indeed, he would go weeks without telling me he had cracked some ribs in a game. It was really only tattoos and sticky tape holding him together at this stage, but I also knew if he made the decision to play, he could and he would. When he put his mind to anything, no injury would stand in the way. I've seen him play countless games with the kind of injuries that would keep most people bedridden, yet he would be out there facing human brick walls on a football field. I have never met a tougher man in my life.

But now that his future was uncertain, that resolve was wavering. Determination cannot exist in the presence of doubt. Mat needed clarity. He mulled over the various factors for several weeks and finally came to a decision.

One sweltering Gold Coast day, we were relaxing in the lounge room while the kids were running round outside, shooting each other with water pistols to keep cool. The day before Mat had played an amazing game against the Parramatta Eels, which the Titans had won.

Mat winced as he reached for the television remote, clearly feeling the pain of some injury from the game. He turned down the volume. 'I'm going to call a press conference.'

'What have you decided?' I asked tentatively, already knowing from his body language and attitude what he would say. He turned to me with a look full of clarity. He knew where he was going now.

'That's it. I'm done.' He said it with an air of utter finality. I loved his ability to make the toughest decisions. It wasn't a quality I possess: I often found it difficult to make decisions of any kind, let alone the really hard ones like this.

A press conference was called at the Titans Centre of Excellence for the next day. Mat had left the house early for training and he would face the press after his first session that morning. I drove the kids to the centre mid-morning so we could all be there to support him. No therapy for Max today — his daddy needed him.

As we drove across the parkway and over the hill, the stadium came into view. It was always exciting to see Skilled Park, the Titans' home ground, on the horizon when we were driving to a game. I wondered if we would ever feel that same excitement again, without the knowledge that Mat was playing there that night.

We pulled up around the side of the building in the car park and hurried inside, trying unsuccessfully not to catch the attention of the throng of media that was arriving for the press call. As the kids' squeals of delight echoed off the solid walls of the building, I felt a dull ache in my head from the nervous bottle of wine I had consumed with the neighbours the night before. I massaged my temples in the lift and hoped to God I would not be asked any questions.

I found Mat reviewing their previous game on a computer, Titans staff milling around him.

'Are you ready to do this?' I asked, a little hesitantly. The last press conference we had attended together had been for the end of his father's life, as I carried our unborn son in my womb in anticipation of a new beginning. Perhaps ironically we were here for another ending that would also give birth to a new beginning.

'Yep, all good,' he responded. There was no doubt in his mind that he was making the right decision, so I took comfort in that certainty. I followed him into the conference room, holding hands with Max and Phoenix.

From the murmurings I heard as the press began filing into the room, I could tell they thought Mat was going to announce he had another year with the club. With his impressive performances on the field of late, I was not surprised. Just weeks earlier he had won them the game against St George, kicking a phenomenal field goal in golden point extra time, right on the buzzer.

Max and Phoenix were sitting quietly, playing games on my iPhone and one borrowed from Kevin Gordon, winger for the Titans. He had snuck in to show his support for a senior player who had been a mentor for him and so many of the other young players.

Coach John Cartwright and CEO Michael Searle settled in on either side of Mat at the table at the front of the room. Every radio and television station in the country had their microphones on the table, all pointed at Mat. He stared at them all, gathering his thoughts for a moment, then cleared his throat and began.

'I've asked you all here today to announce my retirement from the NRL.' A hush fell over the room, journalists looking dumbfounded at one another.

'I feel like I can compete still but I think the time's right to go out,' he added.

The disappointment was evident as journos fired questions from left, right and centre. Mat handled each question and objection with the media-savvy ease you would expect from someone so respected in his field for so many years.

Although Titans fans were devastated by the decision, it was as though a massive weight had been lifted off Mat's shoulders and he began to play some of the best football of his career. He was also so much happier within himself at home and excited to have more time with the kids. He had missed out on so many things due to his sporting commitments that he was really looking forward to doing normal 'dad' things.

In the meantime, however, he had a premiership to win. The Titans were really the team to beat in the competition. They had made it through to the semifinals, playing the Sydney Roosters at Brisbane's Suncorp Stadium. The Titans had organised a bus to take family members up there on the night, so I took Jack and Skyla with me. We were so excited on the bus with the highest hopes, thinking about the win the Titans would have that night, allowing Mat to finish his career on a high. So many NRL players spend their whole careers aiming to win a premiership and never achieve it. Then again, so many achieve it with very little effort, just happening to land on the winning team.

Mat's goal was to win the premiership ring that his father had strived for throughout his whole career and never won. Steve's legacy to Mat was that striving: being the second generation aiming for that elusive ring. This was about more than just a bunch of football games to him: this was about finally realising a dream that their family had reached to grasp for over thirty years.

If the Titans got to the final, then Mat was also going to play his two hundredth NRL game. It all seemed as though it was just meant to be.

Sitting in the stands, we could feel an electricity humming through the crowd. The build-up to the game had been unbelievable. The fans, the press — everyone wanted the 'fairytale ending' for the team and for Mat. All of our neighbours and close friends were there to cheer the Titans on. It was an incredibly emotional time. Watching that game was one of the most stressful things I have ever had to endure, next to my journey with Max in the early days.

I held onto the hope that we would do it, we would win it. I didn't let go of that thought until the last buzzer sounded and the game was over. We had lost.

I began crying uncontrollably, feeling cut to the core as I looked out at my husband and saw the dream of that fairytale ending slowly dissipating into the steaming grass. This was the very last time he would be on a football field. I knew how much it would have meant for him to win this game. I sobbed on the shoulder of my neighbour, who was sitting beside me, and he patted my back consolingly. One part of me couldn't believe that I was getting so emotional over a footy game — the same girl who didn't even know what a try was when I first met Mat.

As Mat did a lap of honour, every fan wanted to touch him, shake his hand, pat him on the back. I hugged Jack as he rubbed a tear from his eye, clearly emotional for his dad. We watched as he was interviewed, putting on a brave smile for the camera. When it was finished, he ran over to us. I leaned over the barricade and embraced him so hard — I didn't want to let go of him. I felt like a lioness trying to shield its cub from harm.

We mourned the bodiless death for several weeks. After that, Mat and I decided it was time to look to the future. I believe that when there is an ending, there is always a beginning: we now had an entirely new phase of life to enjoy together, without a whole team of men to share it with. When I looked at it that way, I for one felt decidedly better.

25

Gaze no more in the bitter glass
The demons, with their subtle guile,
Lift up before us when they pass,
Or only gaze a little while ...

— W.B. Yeats, 'The Two Trees'

Max's fourth birthday had come and gone and he was still not completely out of nappies. Anyone who is a parent will understand the pressure to have a child toilet-trained by a certain age. The older the child becomes, the more embarrassed and inadequate as a parent you can be made to feel. Autism or not, I bet a lot of mothers beat themselves up over the nappy thing.

At friends' houses or on play dates with kids the same age as Max, I was painfully aware that they were not only fully toilet-trained, they could also converse meaningfully with their parents. I know this shouldn't have affected me, I know that every child is different, but as a mother you take a sense of pride in the way your children conduct themselves and by watching their development. Conversely, you feel that people judge you on how your children look and behave — and they do, whether you like it or not. You are the mother, after all, and it is your job to ensure that your children behave appropriately in public.

Although the principle seems to me rather archaic, there is still an unspoken law that the father provides for the family and the mother cultivates, guides and nurtures the children as well as keeping house. There's not a whole lot of equality there, but it is what it is. If you doubt it, think about the last time you saw a child misbehaving in public — were people looking to the mother to sort it out, or to the father? Or what about when you enjoy a beautifully cooked meal at someone's house — was it the man you were most likely to thank, or the woman?

Just as I felt defeated over Max's lack of developmental progress, I would also feel a sense of failure when my house was not clean and orderly. We women place a lot of pressure on ourselves in these areas — well, I do anyway. Even in our house, where Mat contributes equally to these things, I don't think he feels that same sense of failure when the house is not looking up to scratch and the neighbours decide to pop in.

I loved that Mat was strong for me, though. I loved that he was logical. He was the one who could calm me down when I started my emotional self-punishment on all of these seemingly trivial matters.

Max had been refusing to use the toilet for his number twos for too long now — it had to end. He had his routine when he needed to go, and if you tried to tamper with it, all hell would break loose. Max's routine consisted of going to his room, usually around breakfast time, getting the nappy himself and then bringing it to me to put on him. He never used any words. Once the nappy was on he would stand on a chair and push so hard he would go crimson in the face. I always found it strange that he wouldn't want to hide what he was doing; instead he would be on show, standing on a chair at the dining table, watching his cartoons. Many a time an unsuspecting child would be next to him at the breakfast table, watching TV, and not realise what was going on beside them until the scent fouled their nostrils. Weet-Bix suddenly never tasted so bad.

Max's therapists really wanted to help him move onto the toilet as well. At kindy he simply refused to go at all, which meant that he would get very agitated and achieve nothing in his therapy as he spent most of the time concentrating on preventing his bowel movements.

His therapists suggested I cut a hole in his nappy and when he was at the crescendo of his dining room table performance I could whisk him onto the toilet. This could be very messy if my timing was off. God forbid if I got distracted by Phoenix in the other room and Max was left unattended, not realising (or caring) that there was a hole where there should be a nappy. Not a good way to start the day.

When Max was starting his toilet training, Jay at SEDU Burleigh Heads gave me a fantastic DVD called *Tom's Toilet Triumph*. It was a Kiwi cartoon that went into great detail about what's happening and where it should happen. It was hilarious but also very helpful for both Max and Phoenix.

After trying a few different approaches, I put my foot down. It was cold-turkey time — the nappies had to go. So all nappies were removed from the house and underpants bought in their place. Jay had suggested I buy undies with Thomas the Tank Engine on them to make Max excited about wearing them and hopefully deter him from wanting to soil them.

It was a long, hard road. Max refused to go at all for the first few days. He was not cooperating in his therapy and he was extremely moody, as you would expect when you don't empty your bowels for several days.

'Keep going, Chloe, you can do it. We can get through this,' I would encourage myself constantly. It's never easy to watch your children suffer, but deciding how you respond to these situations will help you be a better parent in the long run. I knew if I stuck it out long enough it would work out in the end, as hard as it was to watch. I'm grateful that I was firm: if I hadn't been Max could have been in nappies for a very long time, which does happen with some autistic children.

Come the end of day three, Max was pretty much ready to burst. I sat him on the toilet with my iPhone to play with — and the rest is history.

It's always been interesting observing the differences between Max and Phoenix as they developed. They are only fifteen months apart, but Phoenix is a typically developing child — a typically developing girl child at that. All of the milestones I am still waiting for Max to hit, she is hitting and surpassing at great speed.

One day we were in the car driving to the grocery store. Phoenix and Max were in the back, both strapped into their baby seats. Mat was driving. It was raining outside and as usual, Max was staring blankly at the droplets of rain slowly trickling down his window. He could be amused for hours by water: watching it, feeling it, tasting it. Phoenix, however, was completely uninterested in what was happening outside. She had a Buzz Lightyear doll she was given for Christmas; she and Max were obsessed with *Toy Story* and with Buzz Lightyear in particular. She had Buzz in one hand and a Barbie doll in the other and they were deep in conversation together. Buzz and Barbie, that is.

'Buzz Lightyear to the rescue!' she yelled as Mat tried to adjust his rear-view mirror to see what she was doing. Mat absolutely adored Phoenix. He was so gentle and soft with her, even though she could be so loud and demanding. She comes from a long line of bossy demanding women on my side of the family, so I guess it was inevitable she would fit that mould.

'What're you doing, Buzz?' Barbie asked. Mat glanced over at me as we tried to stifle a laugh with some pretend coughing. Phoenix would become enraged to the point of screaming if she discovered we were laughing at her and not with her.

'Nuffing, what're you doing, Buzz?' this convivial banter would go on and on all the way to the grocery store.

Listening to her rattle on, I began to have a revelation of sorts. This was the functional play I had heard so much about. I had seen countless videos of therapists acting out this style of play, to encourage it in ASD kids. For some reason ASD kids just couldn't do it or understand it; it did not come naturally to them as it clearly did to typically developing kids. The ability to make believe is one of the greatest attributes of a child — one that we as adults admire so much, and often yearn to have again in the same naïve way. My eyes began to fill with tears. I felt suddenly weighed down by an overwhelming mix of emotions, and in my reflection the rain sliding down the window masked the drops sliding down my cheeks. I was feeling immense happiness that my little girl, my angel, was not autistic. She was proving this by her functional play and her advances in other milestones that are not prevalent in ASD kids. But at the same time I felt a deep sadness that from now on, I would always have a gauge of how delayed Max was developmentally.

Just as I had anticipated when Max was at the SEDU, Phoenix would be my perpetual reminder of just how far behind he was. By the same token, though, she was the perfect role model for Max. Phoenix leads him outside his comfort zone all the time; she gives him a consistent example of how he should and could be, and never treats him any differently to any other child she would meet. To her, he is just Max — although she can be quite

262

protective of him too. One day Max was on a slippery dip at the park when another kid climbed up the other way and tried to force him to get off the slide. Phoenix marched up and told the other boy off. Unfortunately she topped it off by hitting him across the head — I don't know where she gets that aggressive streak from.

Even if we failed at everything else, Max would never be pigeonholed or categorised in our house. He was Max and we loved him for who he was, with every little quirk he possessed.

26

I will arise and go now, for always night and day
I hear lake water lapping with low sounds by the shore;
While I stand on the roadway, or on the pavements grey,
I hear it in the deep heart's core.

— W.B. Yeats, 'The Lake Isle of Innisfree'

A year had passed since our inaugural 4 ASD Kids charity weekend, and we were ready to go again. After the success of the first one we had decided it should be a regular event on our fundraising calendar. Apart from anything else, it gave us a great excuse to go back to Sanctuary Cove every year, a place that held so many special memories for us.

This time, though, we were a whole lot better prepared. We had all of the right people in the right places to ensure the event went off well. Phil Harte and Andy Payne had had a dispute of sorts and each had gone their own way. Andy went out on his own and started Limetree Events, taking over the organisation of the 4 ASD Kids event. This would be Limetree's first big event, so a lot was riding on this weekend on so many levels.

264

Second time round we were finding it easier to gain support. Audi came to the party in a big way and gave us a brand-new A1 to give away. Andy came up with the idea of selling off 1,000 gold balls to commemorate Mat's retirement. 'Mat's Golden Balls', as I called them. At $150 each, you got a ball as well as entry into the raffle for a chance to win the car — not a bad deal.

We had a massive team of celebrities attending our second weekend. Charlotte Dawson from *Australia's Next Top Model* and Corinne Grant from *Rove* were there, and Sandra Sully, newsreader, was MCing the ladies' brunch. Matty Johns came along with his family for the weekend; V8 supercar driver Russell Ingall was not only attending but had donated a signed helmet to auction off; Tour de France cyclist Robbie McEwen was there with his family and had donated one of his bikes to auction too. There was no shortage of big names to draw the crème de la crème of the Gold Coast to our little do.

The golf day on the Friday went off without a hitch — almost. According to Mat, he had been driving a buggy on the course with Jack in the back, along with his mate Jake, when it tipped over into a sand dune. No-one was hurt but the owner of the golf buggy was not impressed when it was returned in considerably worse shape than when it had set out in the morning. Mat said he had been reversing over the hill and had not seen the bunker. The paper ran a photo of the upturned buggy, just to add to the embarrassment.

More headlines were to follow, though. During the ladies' brunch the men and the kids went out on the water. Boats ferried them out to McLarens Landing, where they got to eat, drink, be merry and take turns riding on sea biscuits (inflatable rings towed behind a boat) and jet skis. My brunch went extremely well and the ladies had a wonderful morning. Corinne and Charlotte had entertained us and we had seen some fantastic clothes for women and children in the fashion parade. Not to mention drinking champagne for most of the morning.

Because of the early bubbles I had decided to head back to the room to rest before the big gala dinner that night. Max and Phoenix had a babysitter looking after them, while Jack and Skyla had gone out on the water with Mat. I was a bit concerned about Mat getting carried away, as footballers are prone to do when it's an all-you-can-drink affair. The two of us were to host the dinner that evening and so I was nervous that he might be a bit the worse for wear. I had tried calling several times but to no avail, so I decided to lie down for a rest.

After an hour's nap I started getting ready for the dinner. I had just walked in to my hair and makeup artist's room to start the lengthy beautification process when a text message pinged through.

Having the best time this has been one of the greatest days of my life. Love you. Mat

'Great, sounds like Mat's already pretty drunk,' I said to Jodie as I sat down.

She chuckled and began blow-drying my hair. When Jodie had finished with me I went back to my room to work out which dress I was going to wear. As I walked into our hotel room, I realised Mat had still not returned. We were scheduled to have a meeting with Andy and run through the script for the night in half an hour.

'He's cutting it fine,' I muttered angrily and dialled his number on my phone.

'Hello.' His voice came down the line as though he were very far away.

'Talk into the phone, I can't hear you very well,' I said, beginning to lose my patience. 'Where are you?' I added in a rather parental tone.

'We're on the boat on our way back,' he replied, still sounding like he was in a bubble. 'We've had some engine problems so we're travelling back slowly.' I could hear laughter and music in the background. Engine problems — yeah, right, I thought to myself.

'Well, hurry up, we have a meeting in half an hour,' I barked, becoming more and more incensed with how laidback he was sounding.

'Moving as fast as we can.' He hung up the phone.

I made sure I had everything I needed and headed out the door to meet with Andy and go through the proceedings. As I walked over to the Woolshed, the evening hung clear and mild around me. The stillness of the night was breathtaking, yet somehow a little ominous, too.

My pleasure in walking through the evening air dissolved as the reality of Mat not being back muscled its way into my thoughts again. I would be absolutely furious at him when he showed up intoxicated. How selfish to do this today of all days. Silently I worked myself up into a rage; my steps became louder and harder on the pavement as I stormed down to meet Andy.

Regardless of the chaos that could be going on around him, Andy was always calm. It was a trait that I totally admired and utterly lacked.

'Mat's not back yet,' I said grumpily. Andy just nodded. 'What the hell happened to the boat they were on?' I thought.

We sat ourselves down at a table at the back of the room. I had hardly glanced at the decorations when I stormed in but now I was realising just how magnificent the room looked. The ominous feeling began to dissolve as I took in the scene.

'Wow — this looks amazing, Andy,' I said, scanning it from left to right. The tables had beautiful centrepieces and the lighting was dimmed and romantic. A ten-year-old girl called Maddison Brooke was rehearsing on stage. The sound of her voice was evocative and soothing. Limetree had really done an awesome job.

'Let me take you through the rundown,' Andy said, pulling me back to reality.

'I'll just text Mat so he knows where we are,' I said, clicking my thumb over the letters as I spoke. *In the Woolshed with Andy hurry up!* I wrote then pressed send.

Next thing I know my phone rings and it's Mat.

'Hello.' I answered it angrily.

'Darling … I … a … you.' The reception was cutting in and out and again there was that faraway sound to his voice. The phone went dead.

'It's not very good reception in here,' Andy piped up as I stared at my phone in frustration.

I texted him again, my fingers pounding the numbers ferociously.

How bloody drunk are you? We have a dinner to run!

He then texted me back: *I almost died today and so did some others.*

I then texted: *What?*

He responded: *You might need to take the reins tonight.*

'Oh my God. He's bloody drunk!' I was mortified.

Andy looked up from his run sheet, appearing to be slightly concerned at last.

'It's OK, let's just get through this and if I have to do it on my own I will,' I said. Andy continued to run me through everything.

'And I will absolutely kill Mat when he gets back,' I said to myself. This was not on. Of all nights to get loose and leave everything up to me. We had VIP guests to entertain, people to thank. There were going to be around 300 guests there and all of them were expecting to see and talk to the both of us. This was the biggest event of the weekend and Mat was blind drunk! I was furious.

As we were finishing up running through the script, one of Andy's employees came over looking slightly anxious.

'Umm, thought you should know that there's been a little incident on the boat and …'

'Oh great, what now?' I asked mockingly.

'… a few people have got carbon monoxide poisoning,' Andy finished her sentence. He must have known all that time but he didn't want to upset me.

'What?' I shrieked. 'Is everyone OK?'

'They're fine, they're coming to shore with the water police now and they'll be treated by the ambulance out the front,' the young girl finished, clearly shaken by the news she had to deliver.

'Ambulance?' I shrieked again.

'There's one outside — it's just precautionary,' Andy answered.

I excused myself and dashed out to the ambulance. Smartly dressed people were starting to file in to the venue, throwing quizzical looks at the ambulance parked out the front. But there was no-one in there yet, and I had to go back inside and begin welcoming the guests. I shuffled my way back down the stairs, greeting people as I went. I positioned myself at the bottom of the staircase to get the greetings out of the way as soon as possible and go back to check on Mat.

Just as I finished talking to a group of people, a woman tapped me on the shoulder. 'Hi, Chloe, we're from the paper. We have some competition winners here that are ready for their photo to be taken with you and Mat,' she said, gesturing toward some excited punters smiling from ear to ear, then looking around for Mat.

'Um … OK … Mat has been slightly delayed, but when he gets here I'll come and find you,' I said, now stressing about the media finding out about the incident. If they did, it would overshadow everything we were trying to do that night.

My friend Jackie Cross walked up to me. I could tell she knew something was wrong.

'What's going on with you?' she asked straight away. I filled her in on what had happened as best I could and she hugged me.

'You need to forget about all of that right now,' she said. Jackie was very accustomed to hosting big events like this one. She and her husband Billie have run nightclubs on the Gold Coast and in Vegas and were heavily involved in a lot of charity events.

'You have a job to do now. Put a smile on your face and go talk to people.' She kissed me on the cheek and spun me around to the crowd gathering for the dinner. I set to work speaking to people and making them feel welcome, despite the chaotic thoughts that were running riot in my head. Jackie was right: as clichéd as it sounded, the show had to go on.

For the next twenty minutes I chatted with guests as they arrived, listening intently to them. I managed to swipe a champagne off a silver tray without even looking as it went by, which proved a valuable morale booster. Some amazing people were sharing with me their passion for the charity and their stories of lives touched by autism. There really are some remarkable people in the world.

As I finished chatting, I turned toward the staircase just in time to see a slightly dishevelled Mat descending slowly towards me. His face was pale and he looked grim. He had, however, managed to put on his suit and tie. To me he seemed a little shaky on his feet, but hopefully the guests wouldn't notice.

He stopped to greet people as he came down the stairs, the smile on his face strained and slightly forced as he shook hands and exchanged pleasantries. Finally he made it to the bottom of the staircase and I went to embrace him. As I kissed him on the cheek I whispered, 'Are you OK? What the hell happened out there?' We both looked around and smiled at guests. Mat tried to speak loudly enough for me to hear over the hum of the guests but soft-enough that no one else would hear.

'It was like a horror movie, darling. I don't want to talk about it right now.' Mat reached for a glass of water from a silver tray; he caught the eye of some VIP guests and went over to greet them. The show had to go on, I reminded myself.

As I worked my way round the room, some guests said things that made it clear to me they knew something had gone wrong that day. One expressed concern at how intoxicated Matty Johns was when they saw him fall out of a golf buggy on the way up to the party. Matty did have a reputation for enjoying a few drinks, as most footballers do, so I thought nothing of it. Only later did

I find out that he was one of the worst affected and was on his way to the hospital as we spoke.

The doors to the ballroom opened and the guests began to filter through to find their allocated tables. I turned to look for Mat and he was gone. I saw Andy coming towards me.

'Mat's been asked to go to the ambulance for some oxygen,' he said.

'Can I go see him?' I asked.

'Yes, you have time, we won't need you onstage for a little while yet,' he said, patting me on the arm compassionately. I bolted up the staircase as fast as I could in my high heels and ran out to the front of the hotel. I could see the ambulance parked on the far side of the turning circle. I waved at some guests as they moved inside and then ran across the road.

The back of the ambulance was open and inside I could see Robbie McEwen and his son, along with Mat. All three of them were just pulling off their oxygen masks so the paramedics could check their oxygen levels.

'I have to go back in, mate.' Mat was arguing with the paramedic.

'I can't let you go, mate, your levels are not where they should be — you need to go to hospital for further treatment,' the paramedic replied.

'This is really important. This is my charity dinner, I can't leave! All these people have paid good money to be here!' Mat grabbed the oxygen mask; he gestured at a guy standing next to me then pointed at the oxygen valve, asking him to turn it on.

'You can't have any more, mate.' The paramedic was beginning to get agitated as he yanked the oxygen mask out of Mat's hand.

'Darling, just go to the hospital if you need to and I'll handle this.' I was more concerned for Mat's health than he was.

'It's just precautionary, darling, I'm only a little under what my levels are supposed to be.'

Somehow or other he finally managed to talk his way out of the ambulance and we went back down to the dinner. The paramedics would stay there for a few hours, as those guests affected by the carbon monoxide would have to come back during the dinner to have oxygen administered.

Andy was waiting for us at the bottom of the staircase. 'Wait here; we're going to introduce you after the Q and A that's happening right now.'

We stood holding hands at the door, listening to cricketer Damien Martyn and Titans captain Scott Prince banter about Mat. When the Q and A concluded, the MC introduced us.

'And now, please welcome Mat and Chloe Rogers.' We walked into the ballroom, waved and took our seats as though our entrance was always planned this way.

That night we managed to get through all of the speaking we were required to do. The auction had just begun when Mat turned to me and said, 'I think I'd better sneak off to the hospital now.' I nodded in agreement and kissed him on the cheek; he wandered out the door as though he were just going to use the men's room. I did not see him again until nine-thirty the next morning.

We raised $250,000 that night and I drank enough wine to kill a large school of fish. Mat, his fellow Titans player Greg Bird and Matty Johns spent the night in the local public hospital. Matty Johns didn't even make it to the dinner, but his wife took it very well. Her exact words were: 'We're coming back next year and I want to book him back on the carbon monoxide boat because I haven't had to worry about him while he's been in the hospital.' She threw her head back and laughed hysterically; I was so grateful she had a sense of humour about the whole incident.

In fact, everyone was remarkably understanding and recognised that it was just a freak accident. What had happened was that they put up the covers on the boat because of an approaching storm. Once the storm passed no-one thought to open the covers again, so carbon monoxide from the engine exhaust was sucked into the cockpit. No-one on board understood what was going on: people were trying to send messages on their phones but couldn't text, others were feeling ill and falling off their seats. Luckily Robbie McEwen had high-altitude training, so was not as affected and he figured out what was going on.

Later I found out that Mat had actually dived into the ocean to save one of the men who collapsed and fell overboard. He was a hero, and the man in question and his wife could not stop thanking Mat with tears of gratitude in their eyes.

The incident did finally get out to the media. The sporting celebrities had been spotted in the hospital and all of the television and radio channels were calling again. It was too ironic: we had held a press conference to launch our fundraiser and no one showed up, but the minute there was a whiff of controversy every news crew in the country wanted to talk to us. However, we took full advantage of the exposure for the charity. If it meant Mat had to speak about his harrowing ordeal, then so be it. It gave him a double opportunity to talk about our charity and to raise awareness that this sort of boating accident can happen.

On the Sunday, torrential rain set the scene for Sanctuary Cove's annual Christmas Carols concert. *Australian Idol* winner and *X Factor* Australia judge Guy Sebastian was to perform, and despite the weather the turnout was impressive. Mat and I took a golf buggy down to the site; we were amazed at how many people were sitting in fold-out chairs in front of the stage with raincoats and umbrellas as their only protection from the lashing rain.

Mat and I went onstage with our four kids in tow to welcome everyone, then the carols got underway. A fourteen-piece big band performed, the Australian Girls Choir sang, the Special Olympic Dancers made an appearance, and some great local talent took to the stage before the headliner, Guy Sebastian. By the time he came out I had kicked off my stilettos and was dancing around in a poncho with the kids. It was a fabulous night, even though the rain never let up once.

To cap it all off, Mat and Guy picked the winner of the Audi A1 out of a barrel. The winner, Samantha Gleeson, wasn't in the crowd so the boys got on the phone to her. Samantha was ecstatic, but at first she wasn't sure whether it was for real. She hadn't even known there was a car up for grabs: she was just one of Mat's fans and she really wanted a commemorative ball. Her friends had told her not to buy one as they thought it was too expensive, but she went ahead and bought one anyway. The result? A brand-new Audi A1.

After the excitement of giving away the car we invited Guy and his wife and band back to our hotel room for some drinks. Jack and Skyla had stayed in the room watching a movie, as they were not that interested in getting wet down at the carols. When we walked in the door with Guy Sebastian they were pretty excited. Phoenix was particularly thrilled to have a bunch of new people she could show off to and was carrying on as only a three-year-old can, trying to get attention. We were staying in the penthouse at the Hyatt and the room had a grand piano in it. Guy spotted it and immediately sat down and began to play. He truly is a talented musician. Seeing her big chance, Phoenix sat down beside him and began banging on the keys over the top of his beautiful playing. Instead of getting upset, Guy tried to show her how to place her fingers and press the keys with the right pressure. It really was a moment in time.

After a little while I gathered Phoenix up to get her ready for bed. Max was already sound asleep in our bedroom in front of a movie. After I had made sure the children were safely tucked up in bed I came back out into the lounge room, only to find that the group of people I had left there minutes prior had tripled in size. I took a seat to listen to Guy play some of his songs along with some covers on the piano, and before I knew it the room was completely full of people. A lot of people I knew I had not invited. Excusing myself, stepping over bodies and interrupting conversations as I tried to get past, I noticed the front door had been propped open with an old tennis shoe that I did not recognise as ours. So the word had gotten out; there wasn't much I could do but just enjoy the moment — and what an incredible moment it was.

Guy was joined by a crowd of other musicians who entertained us into the early hours of the morning. That debacle of a weekend ended with one of the greatest nights of our life.

27

I have spread my dreams under your feet;
Tread softly because you tread on my dreams.

— W.B. Yeats, 'He Wishes for the Cloths of Heaven'

Christmas, 2010: We had decided to make the trek down to NSW to spend Christmas with my relatives. We had not been back to the Central Coast since that awful time by the campfire when my dad told us he thought Max was autistic. Two years had passed, but I was still nervous about how Max would be this time around. At the same time I was curious to see how my relatives reacted to Max. Some of them had not seen him since then, and he had come so far.

Max had reached a point now where most people who meet him would not necessarily guess he had autism. Sure, there are still a few quirks there: he doesn't always interact with other kids as well as we would like. He's really into grabbing kids at the moment, often in inappropriate places like their bottoms. One day at swimming lessons another boy didn't have a swim top on, so Max kept grabbing him and kissing him on the belly. Not what a typically developed child would do, sure, but he just felt the urge to kiss this lovely fat belly beside him. Maybe it reminded him of his mum's — he always likes to kiss my belly. He's very physically affectionate now, he loves touching skin and the feel of things. I hope as he gets older he might grow out of his desire to grab other kids on the bum and kiss them on the belly.

We flew down to Sydney with all four kids. The flight was uneventful — as it usually is with the kids, except that memorable time with Max. Our good friends Melissa and Gad met us at the airport: they had offered to lend us their eight-seater car, as we hadn't been able to hire a large enough one at such a busy time of year. Slowly we drove out of Sydney through the dense Christmas traffic. As we drove I thought about the last time we were there in the house on the lake. The whole time I was worried about the kids drowning, and kept putting them in front of a movie so I knew where they were. This time I was much more confident: they were very aware of water safety and Max was becoming an exceptionally good swimmer. In fact he's become quite sporty, with excellent hand-eye coordination — that's obviously from Mat's genes.

After several hours crawling along in bumper-to-bumper traffic, we arrived at Ettalong Beach. We had decided to stay in a hotel rather than with family so we could be a bit more independent. The kids loved the hotel, especially the pool —

so much so that they were less than impressed when we had to drag them away to visit relatives. No massive tantrums though, not from Max anyway. He was very much the quiet one now, ironically enough. We hadn't experienced a full-on tantrum from him in public in a long time.

There was one uncomfortable moment at the hotel, though. The morning after we arrived, I woke up and looked out of our window. Dad had organised for us to have adjoining rooms with direct access to the pool. I could see a big group of people gathered, looking down at something. Opening the door to get a better look, I saw a staff member quietly trying to help a duck and her eight ducklings get out of the pool. They seemed to be struggling to get out. The minute I opened the door, Max and Phoenix ran outside to see the duckies.

'Ssshhh!' I breathed to them as we crept closer. Phoenix was walking on tiptoes and even holding her mouth, trying not to breathe so that she could be completely quiet. We got right up close to the baby ducks when Max decided to yell at them.

'Ya ya ya ya duckies!' he bellowed in an irate tone, as if berating them for being stuck. Everyone, including the hotel staff turned to him angrily. 'Sssshhhh!'

I turned bright red, grabbed both of them by the hand, marched back into our room and closed the door. 'Max, that was naughty!' I scolded him. He just stared at the television, watching the early morning cartoons in a trance with a faint smile playing on his lips. He really had no idea.

Later that day, we drove over to the pair of houses that my Aunt Sue and Uncle Ant owned side by side on the bay. My Aunty Jen had flown out from the UK and all of my other aunts, uncles and cousins were there too — all the same people who had looked on sadly as Dad and Jo voiced their opinions about Max two Christmases before. At the time I had wanted to smack them all out, I was so angry. I had thought that they had been judging and talking about my boy behind my back. Now, two years later, I felt a sense of triumph. I was returning to the scene of my humiliation victorious, with a son who could almost now be mistaken for a normal boy.

When we reached Uncle Ant's house the kids took off, bursting with excitement. It was as though they remembered it from two Christmases ago. Loaded down with Christmas gifts for all the kids in my extended family, I went over to greet the throng of relatives. It had been so long since I had spoken to many of them, so I took my time playing catch-ups. Max and Phoenix were safe with the water, I knew, and would not have gone far, so I was comfortable chatting with everyone as I slowly made my way to the house. Just as I had almost finished greeting everyone I heard a piercing scream from behind the house. It was Max. It's funny how when you have kids you get to recognise their cries — and to know what each one means. I can tell when Max is hurt, frustrated, wanting the TV channel changed, or when Phoenix has taken something from him he was playing with. This time I knew he was hurt.

First to come running from behind the house was a little boy I had never seen before. My cousin Emma went over to see if he was OK, and I worked out it was Baz Luhrmann's son. Emma was the film director's nanny and I had been told his two children might be here for the day. Max emerged next, clutching his hand and wailing. We all crowded around him.

To this day I'm not quite sure what happened, but at the time some people believed little William had bitten Max, which is a normal occurrence for kids that age.

'What happened, Max?' I asked him, putting down all of my stuff. 'Was it a doggy?' I probed, as someone had said there was a dog next door.

'Doggy, yes,' he replied. I was happy with that answer and explained to everyone that Max had told me himself it was a dog. More than anything else I wanted them all to know that he had told me, he had spoken. None of them had expected him to be able to explain what was wrong, as last time we were here he could not. I was so proud of him and wanted them to see he had demonstrated his ability to communicate almost as soon as we had arrived.

From the instant you are handed an ASD diagnosis for your child, your mind instantly turns to the worst-case scenario: through your mind run all the horror stories of children smearing faeces on the walls and endlessly banging their heads. The media loves those sensational stories, so that's the image that we are all given. What most people don't realise is that it's called 'the spectrum' for a reason: there are varying degrees of symptoms and abilities.

Later on that day, just before we left, the family were all sitting around having a glass of wine. Max had been quietly playing with Phoenix, when I had asked them if they would like some lemonade. They were both extremely excited at the prospect as I very rarely let them have soft drinks. the two of them almost bowled each other over trying to get to me first. I poured some into Max's glass. He was looking over his shoulder back at all of the family sitting around the table. He seemed to have an idea and made his way purposefully towards everybody.

My aunties and uncles looked up, a little unsure what to expect. Max lifted his glass and looked one of my aunts in the eye. A flicker of concern danced across her forehead until Max rather loudly exclaimed 'Cheers!' and clinked his glass with hers. Everyone erupted into laughter and looked on amazed as he slowly made his way around the table clinking glasses and looking every relative in the eye. Dad would later tell me how that had been a pivotal moment for him realising just how far his little grandson had come. For many people, being on the spectrum makes it harder for them in life, but it is not necessarily the end of their life.

When we left that night my heart was full of pride. Through the course of the day, after he had calmed down, Max had asked for various things he needed or wanted: drinks, chips, the toilet.

My little boy was developing his communication. All of that pain and suffering, the trials and tribulations were beginning to pay off.

Back at home a couple of weeks later, I was organising dinner for the little kids late one afternoon when the phone rang. It was school holidays, and Jack and Skyla had gone down to visit their grandparents on the Central Coast for a few weeks. They were due to fly back in five days time.

'Me get it,' Phoenix screamed, diving for the receiver. I had been mashing vegetables but was quick enough to drop the masher into the pot and grab the receiver before her sticky little hands could get to it.

'Mummy's got it, sweetheart,' I said with a firm smile. She had become passionate about speaking on the phone lately but I was wary of her answering it, as she would often be reluctant to give it up. This was not great if it was work— or business-related — or an emergency, for that matter.

'Hello,' I answered, upbeat despite Phoenix's bottom lip quivering in disappointment.

'Hi, Chloe.' Skyla's familiar voice came down the line. She sounded a little emotional.

'Hi, Bub, how are you?' I pointed to Phoenix and then her chair as if to say, 'Sit down and get ready for dinner.' She turned on her heel and took her bottom lip over to her dinner plate at the table. Max was sitting quietly, watching cartoons.

'Did you get my message on Dad's phone?' she asked, not answering my question.

'No, honey, your dad's in a meeting.' Mat had met with Michael Searle, the CEO of the Titans, to talk about his involvement with the club after retirement. He had been one of the punters' favourite players, so the club was especially keen to keep him involved.

'What was the message, honey?' I asked, slightly worried that something was wrong.

'I've decided … I … I want to come live with you.' A lump formed in my throat. Jack had been living with us for a year now and we were ecstatic to have him. I knew how much this would mean to Mat, but I was also wary that Skyla was only eleven and this was a massive decision for her to make.

Jack had made the same decision when he was her age. Unfortunately lawyers had to get involved in order to make it a reality for him. We spent a lot of money on a custody battle for Jack and we won. We put him into the very best school up here on the coast, which was Mat's old school — The Southport School, or TSS as it's known. But after a semester Jack decided to go back to his mum's. This absolutely crushed Mat. He was depressed for a long time. He doesn't talk so much about his feelings, but when he is emotionally wounded you can see it in his face and the way he holds himself. As a parent, you would always without question go into battle for your child — a father for his son especially. But I can imagine he would feel betrayed after winning the battle, only to have the result reversed by the one for whom you were fighting.

Eventually Jack had come back to live with us again. We had left the door open for him despite what had happened. It was devastating to spend that much money only to have him change his mind; however, we also knew that he was just a child and he wasn't trying to hurt us. He was simply trying his best to keep everyone happy, including his mum. He is a beautiful boy with a massive heart.

I was acutely aware of the possibility of this happening again.

'Really, sweetie? Is this really what you want?' I asked, trying to hide the emotion in my voice.

'Yes, I've spoken to Mum and she agrees — and so do Nan and Pop.'

I had a really good relationship with Michelle's parents, Wayne and Loretta (or Nan and Pop, as the kids referred to them). I understood just how important they were to the kids, so I never wanted them to feel uncomfortable to call at our house or to spend time with them. Loretta and I were able to talk about the kids quite easily together — in fact, it was a lot easier for us than for Mat and Michelle.

Mat would be ecstatic when I told him. We had long imagined us all being together one day and it brought tears to Mat's eyes whenever we spoke of the possibility.

So it was decided: Skyla was coming to live with us. We immediately set to work transforming our little house into a home for six people instead of five. Mat was so excited that his daughter was joining us, he really went all out. He painted the upstairs rooms to make them fresh and inviting and we bought bunk beds for Max and Phoenix. Jack already lived in his teenage den downstairs next to the garage, which he loved.

I wasn't sure how Max would react to sharing a bedroom with Phoenix. All in all, I anticipated a bit of a struggle with him over such a major change. But I needn't have worried: Max was absolutely thrilled to be sharing with Phoenix. He got to sleep in the top bunk and he loved that.

With that hurdle cleared, we were able to focus on Skyla's arrival and consider how well she would be received by everyone else in the house, as well as whether or not she really was here to stay.

Skyla arrived at the airport around 7 in the evening. Mat, Jack and the neighbouring kids had made a sign welcoming her and Mat and our kids had all gone out to the airport together to pick her up in the Audi. Skyla was ecstatic that everyone had made so much effort.

As it turned out, Skyla fitted in extremely well, helping out so much with the little ones. Both of the older children are very protective of Max, especially in social environments when he can get himself in a bit of trouble by saying or doing the wrong thing. Having another female around the house has just been fantastic for me, too, counteracting the 'Testosterone Central' effect that comes with having three males in the family.

Someone else who has thrived is Max. Since all of his siblings have been living together under the one roof his development has accelerated so much. He wants to communicate more with them every day.

One morning I was rushing around, getting everyone ready for school and kindy. Max had been watching one of his favourite cartoons, *The Penguins of Madagascar.* It's a very funny series, based on the penguins from the movie *Madagascar.* Max looked so content, sharing the couch with his two sisters and older brother.

'How are you today, Max?' I asked him. This was one of the social questions I had insisted his therapists work on in his sessions, as it was a question I regularly asked all of our kids.

In one of my fortnightly meetings with his therapists, they told me he had an unusual answer that week. I had been suffering at the hands of a terrible flu virus all week and had only just come good. His therapist Janelle said she had asked, 'How are you today, Max?' To which he replied, 'I feel like shit!' Needless to say I had some apologising to do and since then I've been very wary about dropping the 'S bomb' around him. It's the only swearword I have found terribly difficult to give up.

This particular day, however, Max had a different answer to the one he had been taught — and different to the one he had accidentally been taught by his mum, but this new answer seemed to me very fitting.

'How are you feeling today, Max?' I asked, as I did every morning.

'Living the dream,' he replied with an American accent, sounding just like the penguins in his favourite cartoon.

We all burst into hysterical laughter, and my heart was filled with joy as I realised that he was right. Like most families, we had faced plenty of adversity and our fair share of tribulations. But together we were a unit; together it was us against the world, and together we had decided to face things with hope and optimism. We were happy, we were healthy, our family was supportive and loving. So yes, we really were living the dream. Our dream.

I believe success is in the struggle, not just the end result. Max and I had gone through so much adversity together, but it was our very struggle that brought us out on top. I realise now how important every struggle with my family members had been in order for us to have a stronger bond and unite against this hurdle. The more hurdles we have overcome in life the more lessons we have learnt.

Max is short for Maxwell, his last name is Rogers. His name stands for what he represents, which is a combination of Mat and me and we are a combination of our families. Every day, step by step, together as a family, warts and all, we were winning this battle against autism. If we can overcome, anybody can. Perhaps I had been the right mother for the job after all.

Endnotes

1   Kinney, Munir, Crowley, Miller, 'Prenatal stress and risk for autism', in *Neuroscience and Biobehavioral Reviews*, Volume 32, Issue 8, October 2008, Pages 1519–1532.

2   www.abc.net.au/science/articles/2011/11/09/3360124.htm? site=science&topic=health

3   www.4asdkids.com

Helpful Resources

AUSTRALIA WIDE

Benison O'Reilly and Seana Smith, *Australian Autism Handbook*,
Jane Curry Publishing, Sydney, 2008

www.4asdkids.com — send us an email if you require funding or know
someone whose child does

www.autism.org.au

www.autismspectrum.org.au

www.fahcsia.gov.au/sa/disability/progserv/people/
HelpingChildrenWithAutism/Pages/default.aspx — this is a
particularly helpful page on support and funding, on the website
of the Australian Government Department of Families, Housing,
Community Services and Indigenous Affairs.

www.tonyattwood.com.au

QUEENSLAND

www.abiq.org

www.autismqld.com.au

NSW

www.lizardcentre.com